I0417057

The Menstrual Cramps Cure

Dr. Susan's Healthy Living
drsusanshealthyliving.com

Facebook.com/DrSusanRichards
drsusanshealthyliving@gmail.com
(650) 561-9978

Mention of specific companies or products in this book does not suggest endorsement - by the author or publisher. Internet addresses and telephone numbers for resources provided in this book were accurate at the time it went to press.

ISBN 978-1512213027

Note

The information in this book is meant to complement the advice and guidance of your physician, not replace it. It is very important that any person who has medical problems be evaluated by a physician. If you are under the care of a physician, you should discuss any major changes in your regimen with him or her. Because this is a book and not a medical consultation, keep in mind that the information presented here may not apply in your particular case. In view of individual medical requirements, new research, and government regulations, it is the responsibility of the reader to validate health practices and treatments with a physician or health service.

Table of Contents

Introduction

Dear Friend,

I have written this book just for you, to share with you the all natural treatment program that I have developed and successfully treated thousands of my patients who have suffered from menstrual cramps and pain. As a physician practicing women's health care and preventive medicine, I have worked with many thousands of women who have suffered from menstrual cramps and menstrual pain month after month. Moderate to severe menstrual cramps can really impair a woman's ability to function anywhere from a day to even more than a week each month.

I have been thrilled to see so many of my patients benefit and gain significant relief of cramping and pain with my all natural treatment program. I would like to share with you with the best therapies that natural and alternative medicine has to offer.

Helping so many women gain relief from their menstrual cramps and pain has been a truly wonderful and satisfying experience. In my medical practice, I always emphasize safe and effective natural therapies along with any medical treatments given. I have always wanted my patients to be knowledgeable participants in their own health care program. I have always been impressed with how positively my patients have responded to this approach.

My patients have uniformly communicated to me that they have an intense desire for resources and information on how to stay healthy and free of menstrual cramps. They also understand how important it is for them to take an active role in their own healing process. I personally encountered the need for effective all natural therapies during my own teenage years and throughout my twenties when I suffered from severe menstrual cramps and PMS. It was only after I started my own self-care program that I finally got permanent relief from these problems.

Learning to Cure My Own Menstrual Cramps

My own experience with menstrual cramps was a long and agonizing one. I began to have severe cramps as soon as I started to menstruate as a young teenager. I found very few treatment options available to me as a teen, except for aspirin, a hot water bottle, or simply going to bed and lying there for hours in pain, hoping the cramps would finally stop. Very little information was available on self-care treatments at that time, and I received absolutely no lifestyle information from my physician on the importance of nutrition and exercise in preventing cramps.

My cramps continued to be quite severe throughout college and medical school. As a doctor in training, I had access to the best medical care. I tried every medication possible that might help me including pain pills, muscle relaxants, and antispasmodics, but nothing really helped relieve my symptoms effectively, except on a very temporary basis. I also suffered from PMS during those years, so my menstrual cramps were preceded by days of anxiety, irritability, bloating, and food cravings. It is no wonder that I regarded menstruation with a feeling of apprehension. I still remember episodes of menstrual cramps severe enough to compel me to leave the hospital ward when I was a medical student. I would go to the medical students' on-call room and suffer through the agony of viselike cramps.

Luckily, during my internship year, my situation changed. I was doing my specialty training and spent quite a bit of time reading the new medical research. By chance, I spotted an article on the use of nutrition to treat breast cysts in an obstetrics and gynecology journal. I had never been exposed to the concept of nutrition as therapy before; in fact, it had never occurred to me that what I ate could affect my health status. I was intrigued by the article, which described the successful treatment of breast lumps with the use of vitamins. I began to spend time in the medical library looking for information on the treatment of menstrual disorders through nutrition.

During the next few years, I began to test a simple self-care program on myself. I made some dietary changes, cutting out sugar, saturated fat, and caffeine, which had been the mainstay of my diet. As a busy medical student, I depended on "fast foods" such as cola drinks, coffee, sweet rolls, and pizza to help me stay awake and provide a quick source of energy during busy late nights taking care of sick patients. I started to cut down my junk-food intake, increase my intake of vegetables and fruits. I started myself on a vitamin and mineral program that I put together based on my study of the research in nutritional medicine. I was amazed with the results. My symptoms, which had plagued me for years, began to diminish on a month-by-month basis. My quality of life improved as my symptoms receded in a dramatic way. I began to exercise more regularly and started to learn about and practice stress management techniques. I felt better than I ever had in my life. After following my own self-care program, my symptoms were entirely gone and have never come back.

Learning to Help My Patients

I was my first successful menstrual cramps and PMS patient. In the years since I put together my own treatment program, I have worked with many thousands of women patients who have benefited from a self-care approach. I have spent years researching the use of diet, nutrition, and many other lifestyle techniques that relieve and prevent menstrual cramping and pain. I have also shared with my patients specific acupressure points, stretches, exercises routines, and many stress management techniques in order to help relieve their symptoms and enhance their wellness and quality of life.

My goal with patients has always been to give them the resources to help them become healthier women and then maintain this state through beneficial lifestyle practices. I have been thrilled to see that most of my patients have had significant relief of their menstrual pain and cramping symptoms within one or two menstrual cycles.

Researchers have also made many advances in drug treatment. Today there are medications for menstrual cramps to which I never had access to as a teenager. Many of these treat the symptoms of menstrual cramps at least somewhat effectively for those women who need immediate symptomatic relief. I discuss these medications in my book, too.

How to Use This Book

I feel strongly that any woman interested in self-care should have access to the all-natural menstrual cramp relief program that has been so helpful to my patients through years of medical practice. All of this self-care information is now available in this book, and I hope you will find it as useful as my patients have.

I continue to practice these techniques, too. Preventive health care has had tremendous benefits for me; I am healthier and more productive now than I was as a student. I am continually expanding my own knowledge about self-care and am constantly researching new health care techniques for menstrual cramps.

The menstrual cramp self-care program provides very important information for all women suffering from this problem. I have written the program so that each woman reading this book can select from a wide variety of self-help treatment options that I have included. A treatment plan that utilizes only one method and purports to be the only treatment for menstrual cramps and low back pain will probably work for only a small percentage of women.

In my own medical practice, I have found that results are much better if I individualize a treatment program for each patient. For example, some women feel their best on a high carbohydrate, vegetarian emphasis diet while other women need a more meat-based high protein diet. Both of these types of diets can successfully help to eliminate menstrual cramps, as long as they are high in essential nutrients and eliminate foods that trigger pain and cramping symptoms.

As a result, I have included menus, meal plans and recipes in this book that provide you with both of these dietary options to fit your specific needs!

After seeing so many of my patients become healthier over time, I am a firm believer in the power of self-care. Changing lifestyle habits in a beneficial way gives the body a chance to heal itself. I don't believe that an unfavorable medical diagnosis need be a lifetime sentence of poor health.

Unfortunately, finding information about treatments that really work and are presented in a format that can deliver the relief that you are looking for is not easy to find. I wrote this book so that you could receive the same symptom relief benefits as my patients have.

Besides the essential information on diet, menus, meal plans and recipes, I have included information on the best vitamins, minerals, essential fatty acids and herbs for menstrual cramps and low back pain. Nutritional supplementation is a very important part of an optimal health program for women with these health-care problems.

I have also included programs on stress reduction, exercise, acupressure massage, deep breathing exercises, and stretches that are specifically helpful for symptoms arising from menstrual cramps and low back pain. I have also included a chapter on drug therapies so that you can be fully informed about the most effective drug treatments. Read through the entire book first to familiarize yourself with the material.

The workbook in Chapter 2 will help you evaluate your symptoms, while Chapter 3 is an introduction to the self-care treatment chapters in the book. As you read thought the treatment chapters try the therapies listed under your particular symptoms that most appeal to you. On a regular basis, do those techniques that provide relief of your symptoms. Establish a regimen that works for you and use it every day. This program is practical and easy to follow. It can be used by itself or in conjunction with a medical program. And best of all, it works.

The feeling of wellness that can be yours with a self-help program will radiate out and touch your whole life. You will have more time and energy to enjoy your work, family, and other pleasures in life. Most of my patients tell me that their lives have been positively transformed by following these beneficial self-help techniques.

Love,

Dr. Susan

Part I:
Identifying the Problem

1

What Are Menstrual Cramps

I want to begin your healing program by discussing the common symptoms and causes of menstrual cramps as well as their risk factors. This will help you to better understand your condition you so that you can most benefit from the self-care treatment chapters of my book.

Menstrual cramps, or dysmenorrhea (as physicians call it), are one of the most common health care problems that women suffer from during their reproductive years. It has been estimated that as many as 30 to 50 percent of all women suffer from pain during their menstrual period, with the incidence being highest in younger women, from teenagers to women in their thirties.

In fact, at least 10 percent of younger women have symptoms so severe that they are unable to handle their normal activities. Many women have to miss days of work and important social functions because any movement or activity is too painful. For the first day or two of menstruation, they could only handle bed rest until the symptoms finally pass. This often happened to me during my teens and twenties.

Besides the lower abdominal pain, cramp sufferers can also experience backache, pinching and pain sensations in their inner thighs, bloating, nausea, vomiting, diarrhea, constipation, faintness, dizziness, fatigue, and headaches. For those women who must curtail their activities because of cramps, these problems translate into billions of dollars of lost wages and productivity on the job, as well as a significant decrease in the quality of life for several days each month. It is no wonder that women with moderate to severe cramps regard their monthly period with apprehension and even dread.

Despite the many symptoms and the millions of sufferers, menstrual cramps have been traditionally considered by the medical community to be a "minor" female ailment. Doctors treated women as if the problem were "all in their heads." The problem was either ignored or else treated with powerful painkilling drugs and tranquilizers. Often these drugs had significant side effects and did nothing to alleviate or help prevent the problem on a long-term basis. Luckily, the medical community's interest in menstrual cramps has increased during the past two decades. Researchers understand much more about what causes menstrual cramps on a physiological basis. This has led to newer, much more effective drug treatments, as well as nutritional and other lifestyle-related therapies.

The Normal Menstrual Cycle

It is important to look at the normal menstrual cycle and see how it functions. This background will make it easier for you to under-stand why painful menstruation occurs.

First, understand why we menstruate. Menstruation refers to the shedding of the uterine lining, or endometrium. Each month the uterus prepares a thick, blood-rich cushion to nourish and house a fertilized egg. If pregnancy does not occur and the egg doesn't implant in the uterus, then the body doesn't need this extra buildup of the uterine lining. The uterus cleanses itself by releasing the extra blood and tissue so that a fresh buildup can occur all over again the following month, in preparation for a possible pregnancy.

The mechanism that regulates the buildup and shedding of the uterine lining is controlled by fluctuations in your hormonal levels. It begins each month when luteinizing hormones (LH) and follicle-stimulating hormones (FSH) are released from the pituitary, a gland located at the base of the brain. Once FSH and LH are released into the bloodstream, their destination is the ovaries. The ovaries hold all the eggs a woman will ever have, in an inactive form called follicles. During each cycle, the FSH and LH from the pituitary gland cause one follicle to ripen, and normally one egg is released for possible fertilization. As part of this process, the follicles begin to produce the hormones estrogen and progesterone.

Estrogen reaches its peak during the first half of the cycle as the newly released egg is maturing. Progesterone output occurs after midcycle when ovulation has occurred. Ovulation refers to the production of a mature egg cell.

Besides preparing the egg for fertilization, estrogen and progesterone stimulate the lining of the uterus. During the first two weeks following menstruation, estrogen causes the uterine lining to gradually rebuild itself. The inner mucous layer of glands of the endometrium begin to grow long, and the lining thickens through an increase in the number of blood vessels as well as the production of a mesh of fibers that interconnect throughout the lining. By midcycle, the lining of the uterus has increased three times in thickness and has a greatly increased blood supply.

After midcycle, usually around day 14, ovulation occurs; the egg is picked up by the fallopian tube and continues on to the uterus. The follicle that has produced the egg for that month (graafian follicle) is further stimulated after midcycle by LH and changes into a yellow body, or corpus luteum. It is the corpus luteum that secretes progesterone. Progesterone has further effects on the uterine lining. It causes a coiling of the blood vessels of the lining, which becomes swollen and tortuous and secretes a thick mucous.

If the egg is fertilized, it will implant on the uterine wall and the corpus luteum will continue to secrete progesterone. If no fertilization occurs, the corpus luteum begins to deteriorate and the progesterone levels decrease. The lining of the uterus starts to break down and menstruation begins.

Types and Causes of Menstrual Cramps

There are two types of menstrual cramps: primary dysmenorrhea, in which the pain itself is the main problem; and secondary dysmenorrhea, in which the pain is a consequence of another underlying health problem.

By far the most women suffer from the primary type of dysmenorrhea. This classification breaks down into two subtypes: primary spasmodic or congestive. Primary spasmodic dysmenorrhea is the type most commonly found in young women in their early teens to late twenties. It is more common in women who have never borne children. In fact, childbearing seems to mark the end of the primary spasmodic type of cramps in many women. It is characterized by sharp, viselike pains that are caused by a constriction and tightening of the uterine muscle. Some women also feel these sharp pains in the inner thighs and low abdominal muscles, and some additionally experience feelings of hot and cold, faintness to the point of passing out, nausea, vomiting, and bowel changes varying from constipation to diarrhea. The immediate cause of the cramping is that the uterine muscle and the blood vessels that supply the uterus are tight and contracted. Blood circulation and oxygenation to this area are diminished, so the metabolism of the uterus and pelvic muscles is decreased. Waste products of metabolism, such as carbon dioxide and lactic acid, build up, intensifying the pain and discomfort.

Primary Spasmodic Dysmenorrhea. Primary spasmodic dysmenorrhea has been linked to imbalances in the intricate hormonal system that operates throughout the menstrual cycle. First, medical researchers observed that women who don't ovulate, and consequently undergo only the estrogenic effects on the lining of the uterus, do not experience cramps. Therefore, progesterone needs to be present for menstrual cramps to occur. When cramps occur, the changes seen in the lining of the uterus are typical of those occurring during an ovulatory cycle when progesterone is present.

Pain-free menses without ovulation are typically seen in women at both the beginning and end of their reproductive years, that is, in young teenagers who have just started to menstruate and in women who are transitioning into menopause. There is no evidence, however, that women with cramps actually have low levels of estrogen, or conversely, high levels of progesterone. It may be the interplay between the two hormones that influences the tension and constriction in the uterine muscle and blood vessels.

In addition to the hormones estrogen and progesterone, chemicals called prostaglandins also affect menstrual cramps. These chemicals are found in many tissues in the body, including the uterus, gastrointestinal tract, and blood vessels. There are many different types of prostaglandins, all of which affect muscle tension.

However, not all prostaglandins affect muscles in the same way. The series-2 prostaglandins (specifically the E2 and F2 Alpha), trigger powerful smooth-muscle contractions. An overabundance of series-2 prostaglandins is strongly linked to menstrual cramps and pain. These prostaglandins are also linked to high blood pressure because they narrow the diameter of blood vessels. They can also trigger irritable bowel syndrome since they cause cramping of the intestinal muscles. Not all prostaglandins, however, cause muscle contraction. Others, such as the series-1 and series-3, actually promote muscle relaxation and can help relieve menstrual cramps by preventing the release of the series-2 prostaglandins into the surrounding tissues.

Prostaglandins are derived from fatty acids in the diet. The series-2 prostaglandins that trigger muscle contractions are derived from animal fat—meat, dairy products, and eggs. The beneficial muscle-relaxant series-1 and series-3 prostaglandins are derived from vegetable and fish sources of fatty acids. These fatty acids, called linoleic acid and alpha-linolenic acid, are found predominately in raw seeds and nuts, such as flaxseed or pumpkin seed, and in certain fish, such as trout, mackerel, and salmon.

How we eat can actually determine which hormonal pathway we travel, leading to either muscle tension or muscle relaxation. This is a very good example of how our food selection can determine our state of health. Like progesterone, excessive prostaglandin production is seen only during ovulatory menstrual cycles. Prostaglandin production increases during the second half of the cycle, peaking toward the end of the cycle with the onset of menstruation.

Primary Congestive Dysmenorrhea. The pain that characterizes primary congestive dysmenorrhea is different from that of spasmodic cramping. Congestive symptoms produce a dull aching in the low back and pelvic region, often accompanied by bloating, weight gain, breast tenderness, headaches, and irritability. Unlike spasmodic cramping, these symptoms don't improve with age and, in some women, can worsen with age. Some of the worst symptoms are seen in women in their thirties and forties.

Women with congestive symptoms tend to retain excessive amounts of fluid and salt. Bloat accumulates in the pelvic region as well as breasts; it can cause an uncomfortable, dull aching sensation that makes these parts of the body tender to the touch. Excessive amounts of estrogen can worsen these symptoms, since estrogen increases fluid and salt retention in the body.

An excess secretion of the pituitary hormone ACTH can also worsen congestive symptoms. ACTH stimulates the production of adrenal hormones, which are then sent to the kidneys and cause the kidneys to retain fluid. As a result, women urinate less frequently in the time leading up to menstruation. Once the menstrual period starts, this excess fluid is released. Nutritional factors also influence bloating. High-salt foods should be avoided, since they increase fluid retention.

Food allergies can also contribute to congestive symptoms. Women who are sensitive to both wheat and dairy products (two of the most allergenic foods) can have a premature increase in their congestive symptoms. I have observed this in many of my patients. Other high-stress foods include alcohol, which is toxic to the liver. The liver is responsible for the breakdown of estrogen so that it can be excreted from the body.

Excessive alcohol intake can increase the levels of estrogen in the body, increasing pelvic congestion. Sugar causes constriction of blood vessels, which can worsen cramps; both sugar and alcohol should be avoided in a cramp-relief program. When I put women on a salt-free, dairy-free, and wheat-free diet, the tendency to accumulate bloat decreases, as does the dull, aching abdominal discomfort and low back pain.

Other risk factors can also contribute to both spasmodic and congestive menstrual cramps. These include the following variables:

- Use of tampons may contribute to menstrual cramping in some women. Women who find that tampon use worsens their cramps should switch to sanitary napkins.

- Use of an IUD may significantly worsen the spasmodic type of cramping, and the device may need to be removed if symptoms are too severe.

- Bladder infections can cause symptoms of dull, aching pain in the lower abdominal region. Frequent bladder infections near or during menstrual periods can be a problem for some women.

- Vaginal yeast infections can occur during menstrual periods because of changes in the vaginal pH.

- Childlessness is a risk factor for spasmodic cramping; congestive symptoms may actually be worse in women who have had several pregnancies.

- Lack of exercise and poor posture increases the tendencies toward both types of cramps, since blood circulation and oxygenation is decreased.

- Stress can worsen cramps by causing women to tense their pelvic and low back muscles unconsciously.

Secondary Dysmenorrhea. The result of underlying health problems that can cause uterine and low back pain, secondary dysmenorrhea occurs most frequently in older women, typically in their forties and early fifties. Often, periods will suddenly become painful after years of pain-free menstruation. Secondary dysmenorrhea is much less common than the primary types. Some common causes of secondary dysmenorrhea include the following conditions.

Fibroid Tumors of the Uterus. Fibroid tumors occur when the muscular tissue of the uterus grows excessively. Fibroids can grow very large in some women, enlarging the uterus to sizes seen in pregnancy. If they grow large enough to impinge on the bowel and bladder, or if their growth outstrips their blood supply, they can worsen menstrual cramps. These growths occur most often in women during their reproductive years.

Fibroid tumors are stimulated by estrogen. They may expand in size with the use of estrogen-dominated birth control pills, during pregnancy, or in women who secrete high levels of estrogen naturally. Besides causing menstrual cramps, large fibroids can put pressure on the bladder or bowels, causing urinary frequency or bowel changes. Fibroids can also cause excessive menstrual bleeding and pelvic discomfort to the point of necessitating a hysterectomy. In fact, fibroids are one of the most common reasons for the 650,000 hysterectomies performed each year in the United States. Usually such tumors shrink after menopause because of the decrease in estrogen.

Pelvic Inflammatory Disease (PID). This refers to an infection of a woman's uterus, fallopian tubes, or ovaries. This serious infection must be diagnosed and treated immediately in order to prevent scarring of the reproductive organs and infertility. Symptoms of PID include fever, chills, back pain, a puslike vaginal discharge, pain during or after sexual intercourse, and spotting. When chronic, a low-grade smoldering infection can also cause lower abdominal cramps during menstruation. If untreated, the chronic menstrual pain can necessitate a hysterectomy.

Endometriosis. In this condition, pieces of the uterine lining, or endometrium, implant and grow outside the uterus in other parts of the pelvic cavity. Implants can be found on any pelvic structure, including the fallopian tubes, ovaries, and outer wall of the uterus. They can even become embedded in the intestinal and bladder walls.

These tissues, like the normal lining of the uterus, are responsive to hormonal changes and can bleed with the onset of the menstrual period. Although the bleeding from the uterine lining can leave the body vaginally through menstruation, bleeding from endometrial implants in the pelvis is retained by the body and can cause scarring and inflammation over time. Pain is the most common symptom that arises from this structural damage. Women with endometriosis suffer from pain during menstruation as well as during sexual intercourse.

Treatments for endometriosis vary depending on severity of symptoms, the woman's age, and her childbearing status. Supportive therapy often includes anti-prostaglandin medication such as Motrin and Ponstel. Stronger pain killing medication may be used if symptoms are severe. Pregnancy is actually a treatment for endometriosis, since it relieves monthly menstruation.

In fact, doctors have traditionally recommended that women with endometriosis consider pregnancy to alleviate the problem. Unfortunately, women with endometriosis suffer from a higher level of infertility than the general population because of the scarring and other structural damage that endometriosis creates in the reproductive tract.

In some cases, physicians recommend treatments including the use of birth control pills and other hormonal therapies that inhibit normal menstruation and reverse the stimulation of the endometrial implants. These therapies can be quite effective in reversing the process, but their use requires care because of the many possible side effects that can occur. In advanced cases, endometriosis may culminate in a hysterectomy.

In summary, this chapter has given you information on the different types, causes, and symptoms of menstrual cramps. As you can see, menstrual cramps can arise from a variety of conditions. To identify your specific type of menstrual cramp pattern, go on to the next chapter. Chapter 2 contains a self-evaluation workbook that will help you pinpoint the risk factors and lifestyle habits that contribute to your symptoms.

Types of Menstrual Cramps

Primary Spasmodic Dysmenorrhea	Severe viselike pain, backache, tightening and pain sensations in the inner thighs, nausea, vomiting, diarrhea, constipation, faintness, dizziness, fatigue, headaches
Primary Congestive Dysmenorrhea	Dull aching in low back and pelvis, bloating, weight gain, breast tenderness, headaches, irritability
Secondary Dysmenorrhea	Pelvic and back pain, spotting, pain during or after sexual intercourse, fever, chills, pus-like vaginal discharge, urinary frequency, bowel changes

Risk Factors for Menstrual Cramps

- Use of tampons
- Use of IUD
- Bladder infections
- Yeast infections
- Childlessness (primary spasmodic dysmenorrhea)
- Multiple pregnancies (primary congestive dysmenorrhea)
- Lack of exercise
- Poor posture
- Emotional stress

Part II:
Evaluating Your Symptoms

2

The Menstrual Cramps Workbook

I have developed this workbook to help you evaluate your own symptoms as well as your risk factors that can contribute to menstrual cramps. By filling out the workbook sheets you can easily recognize your vulnerable areas. This will be enable you to focus on the self-care treatments that are likely to be the most helpful and successful in providing you with symptom relief.

While most women with menstrual cramps suffer from the type of pain that can easily be treated by self-care therapies, you will need a medical evaluation if you have menstrual cramps caused by conditions such as endometriosis, fibroid tumors or other issues. More in-depth medical testing for these conditions will need to be done by your physician or caregiver.

First, begin to fill out the monthly calendar of menstrual cramp symptoms, starting today. It is very helpful to make several copies of the calendar. If you can recall your symptoms for the past month, chart these symptoms as well. The calendar will allow you to see which types of symptoms you have, as well as evaluate their severity. This will make it easier for you to pick the specific treatments for your symptoms.

After you have filled out the calendar, turn to the evaluations that follow the calendar section. They will help you assess specific areas of your life to see which of your habit patterns are contributing to your menstrual cramps.

When you have completed the evaluations, you will be ready to go on to the self-help chapters in this book and begin your own treatment program.

Monthly Calendar of Menstrual Cramp Symptoms

Grade your symptoms as you experience them each month

○ None ✓ Mild ◗ Moderate ● Severe

Date _____

DAY OF CYCLE	1	2	3	4	5	6	7	8	9	10	11	12	13	14	15	16	17	18	19	20	21	22	23	24	25	26	27	28	29	30	31
Spasmodic Cramping																															
Viselike pelvic pain																															
Low back pain																															
Pain in inner thighs																															
Nausea and vomiting																															
Diarrhea																															
Constipation																															
Hot and cold																															
Faintness, dizziness																															
Fatigue																															
Headaches																															
Congestive Cramping																															
Dull, aching pain in pelvic region																															
Backache																															
Bloating																															
Weight gain																															
Breast tenderness																															
Headaches																															
Irritability																															
Secondary Cramping																															
Pelvic pain																															
Back pain																															
Spotting																															
Pain during / after intercourse																															
Pus-like vaginal discharge																															
Fever, chills																															
Urinary frequency																															
Bowel changes																															

Risk Factors for Menstrual Cramps

You are at higher risk of menstrual cramps if you have any of the risk factors listed below. Be sure to follow the nutritional, exercise, and stress-management guidelines in the self-help section of this book if you have any of the related risk factors for menstrual cramps listed here. Check each risk factor that applies to you.

Risk Factors

Use of tampons   _____

Use of IUD   _____

Recurrent bladder infections   _____

Recurrent yeast infections   _____

Childlessness (spasmodic cramps)   _____

Multiple pregnancies (congestive   _____
cramps)

Endometriosis   _____

Fibroid tumors   _____

Pelvic inflammatory disease (PID)   _____

Lack of exercise   _____

Poor posture   _____

Emotional stress   _____

Daily use of:

Salt   _____

Animal fats   _____

Dairy products   _____

Wheat   _____

Alcohol   _____

Sugar   _____

Eating Habits and Menstrual Cramps

All foods in the shaded area of the following checklist are high-stress foods that can worsen menstrual cramps. If you eat a substantial number of these foods, or if you eat any of these foods frequently, your nutritional habits may be contributing significantly to your symptoms. Read the chapters on beneficial foods, meal plans, and recipes for further guidance on food selection.

All the foods from avocado to fish are high-nutrient, low-stress foods that may help to relieve or prevent menstrual cramp symptoms. These foods should be included frequently in your diet. If you are already eating many of these foods and few of the high-stress foods, chances are your nutritional habits are good, and food selection may not be a significant factor in worsening your menstrual cramps. You may want to look carefully at the stress management and exercise chapters. The activities contained in these chapters may be very helpful in relieving your cramps.

Eating Habits Checklist

Check the number of times you eat the following foods.

Foods That Increase Symptoms

Foods	Never	1x a Month	1x a Week	>1x a Week
Coffee				
Cow's milk				
Cow's cheese				
Butter				
Yogurt				
Eggs				
Chocolate				
Sugar				
Alcohol				
White bread				
White noodles				
White-based flour				
Pastries				
Added salt				
Bouillon				
Commercial salad dressing				
Catsup				
Black tea				
Soft drinks				
Hot dogs				
Ham				
Bacon				
Beef				
Lamb				
Pork				

Foods That Decrease Symptoms

Foods	Never	1x a Month	1x a Week	>1x a Week
Avocado				
Green Beans				
Beets				
Broccoli				
Brussels sprouts				
Cabbage				
Carrots				
Celery				
Collard greens				
Cucumbers				
Eggplant				
Garlic				
Horseradish				
Kale				
Legumes				
Lettuce				
Mustard greens				
Okra				
Onions				
Parsnips				
Peas				
Potatoes				
Radishes				
Rutabagas				
Spinach				
Squash				
Sweet potatoes				
Tomatoes				
Turnips				
Turnip greens				
Yams				
Brown rice				
Millet				
Barley				
Oatmeal				
Buckwheat				
Rye				
Raw flaxseeds				
Corn				

Raw pumpkin seeds				
Raw sesame seeds				
Raw sunflower seeds				
Raw almonds				
Raw filberts				
Raw pecans				
Raw walnuts				
Apples				
Bananas				
Berries				
Pears				
Seasonal fruits				
Corn oil				
Flax oil				
Olive oil				
Sesame oil				
Safflower oil				
Eggs				
Poultry				
Fish				

Exercise Habits and Menstrual Cramps

Exercise helps prevent menstrual cramps by relaxing muscles and promoting better blood circulation and oxygenation to the pelvic area. It can also help reduce stress and relieve anxiety and upset. If your total number of exercise periods per week is less than three, you will probably be more prone to cramp symptoms. See the chapters on the various kinds of exercise that can help relieve and prevent symptoms.

If you are exercising more than three times a week, keep doing your exercises; they are probably making your symptoms less severe. You may want to add specific corrective exercises to your present regimen, choosing them to fit your individual symptoms. There are many options available in the chapters on exercise, stretches, and acupressure massage.

Exercise Checklist

Check the frequency with which you do any of the following:

Exercise	Never	1x a Month	1x a Week	>1x a Week
Walking				
Running				
Dancing				
Swimming				
Bicycling				
Tennis				
Stretching				

Stress and Menstrual Cramps

If you are experiencing any of the following life events, check those that apply to you.

Checking many items in the first third of this scale indicates major life stress and a possible vulnerability to serious illness. In other words, the more items checked in the first two thirds, the higher your stress quotient. Do everything possible to manage your stress in a healthy way. Eat the foods that provide a high-nutrient/low-stress diet, exercise on a regular basis, and learn the methods for managing stress given in the chapter on stress reduction and deep breathing.

If you check fewer items, you are probably at lower risk for illness. Because stresses too minimal to include in this evaluation may also play a part in increasing your menstrual cramps, you will still benefit from practicing the methods outlined in the chapter on stress reduction. Stress management is very important in helping you to gain control over your level of muscle tension.

Check if this stressful event applies to you.

Life Events

_____ Death of spouse or close family member

_____ Divorce from spouse

_____ Death of a close friend

_____ Legal separation from spouse

_____ Loss of job

_____ Radical loss of financial security

_____ Major personal injury or illness (gynecologic or other cause)

_____ Future surgery for gynecologic or other illness

_____ Beginning a new marriage

_____ Foreclosure of mortgage or loan

_____ Lawsuit lodged against you

_____ Marriage reconciliation

_____ Change in health of a family member

_____ Major trouble with boss or co-workers

_____ Increase in responsibility—job or home

_____ Learning you are pregnant

_____ Difficulties with your sexual abilities

_____ Gaining a new family member

_____ Change to a different job

_____ Increase in number of marital arguments

_____ New loan or mortgage of more than $100,000

_____ Son or daughter leaving home

_____ Major disagreement with in-laws or friends

_____ Recognition for outstanding achievements

_____ Spouse begins or stops work

Begin or end education

_____ Undergo a change in living conditions

_____ Revise or alter your personal habits

_____ Change in work hours or conditions

_____ Change of residence

_____ Change your school or major in school

_____ Alterations in your recreational activities

_____ Change in church or club activities

_____ Change in social activities

_____ Change in sleeping habits

_____ Change in number of family get-togethers

_____ Diet or eating habits are changed

_____ You go on vacation

_____ The year-end holidays occur

_____ You commit a minor violation of the law

Major life stress can have a significant impact on the symptoms of menstrual cramps as well as other health problems. It is helpful to assess your own level of stress to see how it may be impacting your health. One popular tool is the Holmes and Rahe Social Readjustment Rating Scale, which was adapted for women and identifies events that cause stress.

Daily Stress Evaluation

This evaluation is a very important one for women with a tendency toward menstrual cramps. Not all stresses have a major impact on our lives, as do death, divorce, or personal injury. Most of us are exposed to a multitude of small life stresses on a daily basis. The effects of these stresses are cumulative and can be a major factor in triggering muscle tension in the pelvic area on an unconscious basis.

Check each item that seems to apply to you.

Work

____ **Too much responsibility.** You feel you have to push too hard to do your work. There are too many demands made of you. You feel very pressured by all of this responsibility. You worry about getting all your work done and doing it well.

____ **Time urgency.** You worry about getting your work done on time. You always feel rushed. It feels like there are not enough hours in the day to complete your work.

____ **Job instability.** You are concerned about losing your job. There are layoffs at your company. There is much insecurity and concern among your fellow employees about their job security.

____ **Job performance.** You don't feel that you are working up to your maximum capability due to outside pressures or stress. You are unhappy with your job performance and concerned about job security as a result.

____ **Difficulty getting along with co-workers and boss.** Your boss is too picky and critical. Your boss demands too much. You must work closely with co-workers who are difficult to get along with.

____ **Understimulation.** Work is boring. The lack of stimulation makes you tired. You wish you were some-where else.

____ **Uncomfortable physical plant.** Lights are too bright or too dim; noises are too loud. You're exposed to noxious fumes or chemicals. There is too much activity going on around you, making it difficult to concentrate.

Spouse or Significant Other

_____ **Hostile communication.** There is too much negative emotion and drama. You are always upset and angry. There is not enough peace and quiet.

_____ **Not enough communication.** There is not enough discussion of feelings or issues. You both tend to hold in your feelings. You feel that an emotional bond is lacking between you.

_____ **Discrepancy in communication.** One person talks about feelings too much, the other person too little.

_____ **Affection.** You do not feel you receive enough affection. There is not enough holding, touching, and loving in your relationship. Or, you are made uncomfortable by your partner's demands.

_____ **Sexuality.** There is not enough sexual intimacy. You feel deprived by your partner. Or, your partner demands sexual relations too often. You feel pressured.

_____ **Children.** They make too much noise. They make too many demands on your time. They are hard to discipline.

_____ **Organization.** Home is poorly organized. It always seems messy; chores are half-finished.

_____ **Time.** There is too much to do in the home and never enough time to get it all done.

_____ **Responsibility.** You need more help. There are too many demands on your time and energy.

Your Emotional State

____ **Too much anxiety.** You worry too much about every little thing. You constantly worry about what can go wrong in your life.

____ **Victimization.** Everyone is taking advantage of you or wants to hurt you.

____ **Poor self-image.** You don't like yourself enough. You are always finding fault with yourself.

____ **Too critical.** You are always finding fault with others. You always look at what is wrong with other people rather than seeing their virtues.

____ **Inability to relax.** You are always wound up. It is difficult for you to relax. You are tense and restless.

____ **Not enough self-renewal.** You don't play enough or take enough time off to relax and have fun. Life isn't fun and enjoyable as a result.

____ **Feeling of depression.** You feel blue, isolated, and tearful. You feel a sense of self-blame and hopelessness. Fatigue and low energy are problems.

____ **Too angry.** Small life issues seem to upset you unduly. You find yourself becoming angry and irritable with your husband, children, or clients.

Read over the day-to-day stress areas that you find difficult to handle. How many items have you checked? Becoming aware of them is the first step toward lessening their effects on your life. Methods for reducing them and helping your body to deal with them are given in the chapter on stress reduction.

How Stress Affects Your Body

This evaluation should help you become aware of where stress localizes in your body. Each woman accumulates stress in a different way, tensing and contracting different sets of muscles in a pattern that is unique to her. This accumulation increases your level of fatigue and lowers your energy and vitality. Storing tension in the low back and pelvic area can worsen cramps, while storing it in the neck can cause headaches.

Check the places where tension most commonly localizes in your body.

____   Low back
____   Pelvic area
____   Stomach muscles
____   Thighs and calves
____   Chest
____   Shoulders Arms
____   Neck and throat
____   Headache
____   Grinding teeth
____   Eyestrain

Part III:
Finding the Solution

3

The Menstrual Cramps Program

I am thrilled that you are now ready to being your treatment program! The self-care chapters of this book will be very helpful in providing you with the relief and healing that you are looking for. I am certain that these healing resources will be as beneficial for you as they have been for so many of my patients as well as myself. In the chapters that follow, you will find wonderful self-care resources. These include my dietary and nutritional supplements program, menus, meal plans and delicious recipes. I have also included chapters on my stress reduction, exercise, acupressure points and stretching programs

There are two ways that you can work with the treatment chapters. You can either begin by going to the chapters that most appeal to you and work with those therapies, first. However, I do recommend that you start right away by reading the dietary and nutritional supplement chapters, no matter what other chapters you work with. The menstrual cramp relief diet and the therapeutic nutritional supplement program are essential to successfully eliminating your menstrual pain and cramping symptoms.

You can also read straight through the rest of the book, get a general overview of the various approaches, and find those you are interested in trying. In doing the exercises in the stress reduction, stretching or other chapters, I recommend that you choose the exercises that are focused on your combination of symptoms. Establish the regimen that works for you and use it each month. Whichever way you choose to approach the treatment chapters, if you follow the program faithfully, you will begin to see great improvements in your symptoms very quickly— often within a month or two. My program should also support your general health and well-being. Many of my patients have been thrilled that they have also enjoyed more energy, vitality, clarity of mind and resistance to illness by following these recommendations.

4

Dietary Principles for Menstrual Cramps

A healthy diet is the cornerstone of a good menstrual cramp self-care program. In fact, I have found that good nutritional habits bring more relief from cramps than any other single factor. Even women who have severe cramps and have used many strong drugs to suppress their symptoms benefit greatly from a proper anti-cramp diet. I have been very impressed by how many women have reported a noticeable decrease in their pain and discomfort within one or two menstrual cycles after starting my program.

Besides the specific benefits these dietary principles will have on your cramps, they will also aid your general health and well-being. Many women have reported that they have more energy and a greater sense of well-being than they have had in years. Often they tell me that symptoms they never associated with their menstrual cramps, such as allergies, frequent colds, sinusitis, nasal congestion and general poor digestive function have cleared up, too.

In this chapter, I discuss in detail which foods worsen menstrual cramps and should be avoided. This list may surprise you, because it contains not only foods that are stressful to the body and are often called "junk foods," but also many foods that are staples of the American diet. Many women eat a diet that they mistakenly think is healthy, not realizing that their food selection is actually contributing to their cramps. Luckily, the list of foods that help to relieve and prevent menstrual cramps is a long one.

Once you shift to a diet of more healthful foods, you will find that they are just as delicious, convenient, and easy to prepare as the foods you are eating now. The information on these foods is the result of years of work with women who came to me with menstrual cramps and had significant relief of their symptoms. I hope you will experience the same great results.

Foods That Help Treat or Prevent Menstrual Cramps

You should emphasize in your diet the foods listed in this section. They provide the range of nutrients you need to prevent menstrual cramps and the many associated symptoms that can occur several days or more each month. Although your symptoms are limited to the days preceding menstruation and its onset, these foods should form the mainstay of your diet throughout the entire month. A poorly chosen high-stress diet during your symptom-free time will increase the severity of your symptoms when menstruation starts.

Whole Grains. I strongly recommend the use of whole grains such as millet, oats, and rice. Many women also tolerate 100 percent rye. These grains are excellent sources of magnesium, which helps reduce neuromuscular tension and thereby decrease menstrual cramps. They are also fairly high in calcium, which also relaxes muscle contractions. They are excellent sources of potassium, as is buckwheat. Potassium has a diuretic effect on the body tissues and helps reduce bloating. Excessive fluid retention is one of the main causes of the congestive symptoms seen with cramps, characterized by dull, aching pain.

Women with cramps may want to avoid eating wheat. This probably comes as a surprise to you because wheat is a mainstay of the American diet. However, wheat contains a protein called gluten that is difficult to digest and can be highly allergenic. In many of my patients with cramps, wheat has worsened fatigue, depression, bloating, constipation, diarrhea, and intestinal cramps. You may want to try a wheat-free diet to see if you feel better after wheat is eliminated. If you have more severe gluten intolerance or food allergies, you may want to eliminate oat and rye also, since they also contain some gluten. You may find that you feel best using buckwheat, corn, and rice. Even these grains should be rotated and used only every few days by women who have food allergies and menstrual cramps.

Another benefit of whole grains is their fiber or bran content. Bran can help reduce the congestive symptoms of cramps since it produces bulkier stools with a higher water content; this helps to get rid of excess fluid in the body. Fiber is also helpful in eliminating the digestive symptoms that occur with cramps. It has a normalizing effect on the bowel movements, helping prevent both constipation and diarrhea. Besides removing excessive water from the body, whole grains appear to help bind fat and remove it from the body, as well as helping lower cholesterol. Oat and rice bran are particularly good for this purpose. Because cancer of the breast, uterus, ovaries, and colon are linked to a diet high in animal fats, the use of whole grains may actually have a protective effect in preventing the development of these diseases.

Whole grains have other benefits, too. They are an excellent source of B-complex vitamins and vitamin E. These nutrients can help combat the fatigue and depressive symptoms seen with the onset of menstruation. They are also an excellent source of protein, particularly when combined with beans and peas.

Whole Grain Cereals. Puffed millet, unsweetened granola, puffed corn, and puffed rice are available as cold breakfast cereals. Cream of rye and buckwheat groats are also good sources of iron. These products can be found in health food stores. Your best bet if you shop in a supermarket is the slow-cooking, old-fashioned Quaker Oats (the quick-cooking kind is a refined grain product and should be avoided). Health food stores offer a wider choice of iron-rich cereals.

Whole Grain Breads. Health food stores offer many different gluten-free whole grain breads including those made of rice, millet, soy-potato, and tapioca flour. Choose brands made without added sugar.

Whole Grain Crackers. Many types of rice crackers are available in grocery stores. Brown rice flour is a good source of minerals. Crackers can be used for snacks or open-face sandwiches. Brown rice cakes are particularly good served with soy spreads, tuna salad, or fruit and nut spreads.

Whole Grain Pancakes. You can make pancakes with buckwheat, rice or oat flour. Concentrated sweeteners such as maple syrup, honey, and applesauce can be used in small amounts.

Pasta. Pasta made of buckwheat, rice, corn, or soy is readily available in health food and ethnic food stores. These types of pasta are easy to digest for women who get digestive symptoms and bloating with menstruation.

Legumes. Beans and peas are excellent sources of calcium, magnesium, and potassium. I highly recommend their use in an anti-cramp diet. Especially good sources of these nutrients include tofu, black beans, pinto beans, kidney beans, chickpeas, lentils, lima beans, and soybeans. These foods are also high in iron and tend to be good sources of copper and zinc. Legumes are very high in B-complex vitamins and vitamin B6, all necessary nutrients for the relief and prevention of cramps and menstrual fatigue. They are also excellent sources of protein and provide all the essential amino acids when eaten with grains. (Good examples of grain and legume combinations include meals such as beans and rice, or corn bread and split pea soup.) Legumes provide an excellent and easily utilized source of protein and can be used as a substitute for meat.

As with grains, legumes are an excellent source of fiber and can help normalize bowel function. They digest slowly and can help to regulate the blood sugar level, a trait they share with whole grains. As a result, they are an excellent food for women with diabetes or blood sugar imbalances. Some women find that gas is a problem when they eat beans. You can minimize this by using digestive enzymes, such as hydrochloric acid, and eating beans in small quantities.

Vegetables. These are outstanding foods for all menstrual cramp symptoms. Many vegetables are high in calcium, magnesium, and potassium, which help relieve and prevent the spasmodic symptoms of cramps. Besides helping to relax tense, irritable muscles, these minerals also calm and relax emotions. Both calcium and magnesium act as natural tranquilizers, a real benefit for women suffering from menstrual pain, discomfort, and irritability. Potassium aids in relieving the symptoms of congestive dysmenorrhea by reducing fluid retention and bloating. Some of the best sources for these minerals include Swiss chard, spinach, broccoli, beet greens, mustard greens, sweet potatoes, kale, potatoes, peas, and green beans. These vegetables are also high in iron, which may help to reduce cramps.

Many vegetables are high in vitamin C, which helps to increase capillary permeability and facilitate the flow of essential nutrients into the tight muscles as well as the flow of waste products out. Vitamin C is an important anti-stress vitamin because it is needed for healthy adrenal hormonal production (the adrenals are glands that help us deal with stress). Vitamin C is also important for immune function and wound healing. Its anti-infectious properties may help to reduce the tendency toward bladder and vaginal infections, which can cause secondary dysmenorrhea. Vegetables high in vitamin C include Brussels sprouts, broccoli, cauliflower, kale, peppers, parsley, peas, tomatoes, and potatoes.

Fruits. Fruits contain a wide range of nutrients that can benefit menstrual cramps. Like many vegetables, fruits are an excellent source of vitamin C, which is important for healthy blood vessels and blood circulation into the tense pelvic muscles. Almost all fruits contain some vitamin C, with the best sources including berries, oranges, grapefruits, and melons. These fruits are also good sources of bioflavonoids, another essential nutrient that affects blood vessel strength and permeability.

Certain fruits are also excellent sources of calcium and magnesium; you can eat them often for your mineral needs. These include dried figs, raisins, blackberries, bananas, and oranges. Figs, raisins, and bananas are also exceptional sources of potassium, so should be eaten by women with fatigue and bloating. All fruits are an excellent source of potassium.

Eat fruits whole to take advantage of their high fiber content. This fiber content helps prevent constipation and the other digestive irregularities frequently seen with menstrual cramps.

Fresh and dried fruits are excellent snack and dessert substitutes for cookies, candies, cakes, and other foods high in refined sugar. Although fruit is high in sugar, its high fiber content helps to slow down absorption of the sugar into the blood circulation and thereby helps to stabilize the blood sugar level. I recommend, however, using fruit juices in small quantities. Fruit juice does not contain the bulk or fiber of the whole fruit. As a result, it acts more like table sugar and can destabilize your blood sugar level in a dramatic manner when used to excess. In this case, less is better. If you want to have fruit juice on a more frequent basis, mix it half-and-half with water.

Seeds and Nuts. Many seeds and nuts are excellent sources of the two essential fatty acids, linoleic acid and alpha-linolenic acid. These provide the raw materials your body needs to produce the muscle-relaxant prostaglandin hormones. Adequate levels of essential fatty acids in your diet are very important in treating and preventing muscle cramps; they are also beneficial for your skin and hair. The best sources of both fatty acids are raw flaxseeds, chia seeds and hempseeds. Other seeds, such as sesame and sunflower seeds, are excellent sources of linoleic acid alone.

Seeds and nuts are excellent sources of the B-complex vitamins and vitamin E, which are important anti-stress factors for women with cramps. These nutrients also help to regulate hormonal balance. Seeds and nuts are very high in other essential nutrients that women with menstrual cramps have a strong need for, including magnesium, calcium, and potassium. Particularly good to eat are sesame seeds, sunflower seeds, pistachios, pecans, and almonds. Because they are very high in calories, they should be eaten in small amounts.

The oils in seeds and nuts are very perishable, so exposure to light, heat, and oxygen should be avoided. Try to eat them raw, and remove them yourself from their protective shells. Seeds and nuts should be eaten raw and unsalted to get the benefit of their essential fatty acids and to avoid the negative effects of too much salt. If you buy them already shelled, they should be refrigerated so their oils don't become rancid. Seeds and nuts make a wonderful garnish on salads, vegetable dishes, and casseroles and can be eaten as a main source of protein with snacks and light meals.

Poultry and Fish. I generally recommend eating meat in moderation. Particularly good are omega-3 fatty acid containing fish like salmon, trout, tuna, halibut, and mackerel. Fish should be eaten no more than once or twice a week due to the high mercury content in most fish. Also good are free range poultry, organic lean red meat and game meat. Fatty cuts of red meats like beef, pork, and lamb should be avoided. This is because they contain the saturated fats that the body uses to produce the series-2 prostaglandins, the hormone like chemicals that trigger muscle contraction and constriction in blood vessels; thereby worsening cramps omega-3 fatty acids are converted within the body to the beneficial series-3 prostaglandins which help to reduce menstrual cramps. I have also found that fish oil capsules, when used as a nutritional supplement, are very helpful for my patients especially when you are eating foods like poultry, eggs and vegetarian diets that lack omega-3 fatty acids.

Instead of using meat as your only or primary source of protein, I recommend that you increase your intake of grains, beans, and raw seeds and nuts, which contain protein as well as many other important nutrients. For many years I have recommended to my patients that they use meat more as a garnish and a flavoring for casseroles, stir-fries, and soups. I also recommend that you buy meat from organic or free range sources—this meat has undergone much less exposure to pesticides, antibiotics and hormones. If you find meat difficult to digest, you may be deficient in hydrochloric acid, a digestive enzyme normally found in the stomach. Try taking a small amount of hydrochloric acid with every meat-containing meal to see if your digestion improves.

Oils. You can use vegetable oils in small amounts for cooking, stir-frying, and sautéing; select oils such as soybean oil and corn oil that contain vitamin E. Vitamin E is an important nutrient in reducing the mood symptoms, fatigue, and cramps that occur at the onset of menstruation in many women. Medical studies show that vitamin E may help to regulate the estrogen/progesterone ratio. This is important because high levels of estrogen stimulate the growth of secondary causes of menstrual pain and cramping like endometriosis and fibroid tumors.

Women with menstrual cramps should take vitamin E in both supplemental form and dietary sources such as wheat germ oil. In fact, wheat germ oil contains the highest levels of vitamin E and is the source for most natural vitamin E sold on the market today. Oils should be cold-pressed because this helps ensure freshness and purity. Keep your oils refrigerated to avoid rancidity.

Foods to Avoid with Menstrual Cramps

If you have menstrual cramps, you should avoid or use only in limited amounts the foods described in this section, because they can increase your monthly symptoms. You will also notice that some of these food are generally recognized as being high-stress, unhealthy foods for the body.

Dairy Products. Dairy products are a high-risk food for women with menstrual cramps. This is always a surprise to many women, because dairy products have traditionally been considered as one of the four basic food groups, and most women use them as staples in their diet, consuming large amounts of cheese, yogurt, milk, and cottage cheese. Yet, dairy products are the main dietary source of arachidonic acid, the fat that your body uses to produce the muscle-contracting series-2 prostaglandins.

I have seen the severity of menstrual cramps decrease by as much as one-third to one-half within one menstrual cycle when women completely eliminate dairy products from their diet. The high saturated-fat content of dairy products is a risk factor for promoting excess estrogen levels in the body. Excessive estrogen is a trigger for endometriosis and fibroid tumors, which are common causes of secondary dysmenorrhea. Also, the high salt content of dairy products increases the bloating and fluid retention of congestive dysmenorrhea.

Dairy products have many other unhealthy effects on a woman's body. The tryptophan in milk has a sedative effect that increases fatigue, a real problem for some women the first day or two of their periods. Many people are allergic to dairy products or lack the enzymes to digest milk. The result can be digestive problems like bloating, gas, and bowel changes, which intensify with menstruation. Intolerance to dairy products can hamper the absorption and assimilation of the calcium they contain. Dairy products have also been shown in clinical studies to decrease iron absorption in anemic women.

Because dairy products are a risk factor for cramps, women who have depended on dairy products for their calcium intake naturally wonder about what alternative sources to use. Women who are concerned about their calcium intake can use the many other good dietary sources of this essential nutrient. These include beans, peas, soybeans, sesame seeds, soup stock made from chicken or fish bones, and green leafy vegetables. For food preparation, potato milk, soy milk, and nut milk are excellent substitutes. You can also use a supplement containing calcium, magnesium, and vitamin D to make sure your intake is sufficient. Nondairy milks are readily available at health food stores.

Wheat and Gluten-Containing Grains. While consuming whole grains has many health benefits, some women with menstrual cramps and other conditions like PMS may find that they are allergic to or intolerant of wheat. Most women are surprised by this discovery, since wheat is one of the staples of our culture and is eaten by most people at almost every meal. However, wheat contains a protein called gluten, which is highly allergenic and difficult for the body to break down, absorb, and assimilate. Women with wheat intolerance are prone to fatigue, depression, sinusitis, allergies, bloating, intestinal gas, and bowel changes.

It can also affect hormonal health and worsen estrogen dominance, aggravating menstrual cramps and other conditions like PMS. In my clinical practice, I have observed how wheat (along with other foods) can trigger emotional symptoms and fatigue in PMS patients, especially during the week or two before the onset of menses.

If you suffer from any of these conditions, you should probably eliminate wheat from your diet and use the many gluten-free breads, breakfast cereals, bagels, English muffins, cookies and other flour based foods that are readily available in health food stores and many supermarkets. Oats and rye, which also contain gluten, should be eliminated along with wheat if your symptoms are moderate to severe.

I have found over the years that the least stressful grain for women with conditions like menstrual cramps and PMS are grains like brown rice, millet, quinoa, wild rice, amaranth and buckwheat. Gluten-free oats are available in health food stores and some supermarkets.

Buckwheat is not commonly eaten in our culture, so most women never develop an intolerance to it. Also, it is not in the same plant family as wheat and other grains. Other infrequently used grains such as wild rice, quinoa, and amaranth should be tried as well. These are available in health food stores in breads, crackers, pastas and cereals.

Whole grass and whole grain flours can be prepared in a variety of ways, including whole grain cereals, breads, crackers, pancakes, waffles, and pastas. They can also be sprouted and eaten raw. A wide variety of these grains and products are available both in supermarkets and natural food stores.

Fats. Like dairy products, the use of saturated fats (which generally come from animal sources, though also from a few vegetable sources, such as palm oil) can intensify menstrual cramps through stimulating the production of the muscle-contracting prostaglandins. In the typical American diet, 40 percent of the calories come from fat. Most of this fat is from sources such as dairy products and red meat. This diet also tends to promote fibroid tumor growth and heavy menstrual flow in susceptible women, because excessive saturated fat intake is stressful to the liver and helps to increase excess estrogen levels. Fibroids can worsen cramps when they grow to be too large, cutting off their own blood supply and pressing on the bladder and intestines.

Saturated fat, primarily from animal sources, also puts women at high risk for heart disease and cancer of the breast, uterus, and ovaries. Women on a high-fat diet also tend to accumulate excess weight more easily. Instead of foods high in saturated fat, eat more fruits, vegetables, grains, fish, and poultry. As often as possible, eat fresh and homemade foods prepared with a minimum of fats and oils. If you must eat packaged and processed foods, read the labels. Avoid those with a high fat content. Red meat should be used only in small amounts. Avoid recipes that use large amounts of butter, cream, cheese or other high-fat food in the preparation.

Instead, flavor foods with garlic, onions, herbs, lemon juice, or a little olive oil (a monosaturated fat that doesn't increase your cholesterol level). Eat raw seeds and nuts rather than cooked ones (cooking alters the nature of the oils), and use them sparingly because of their high fat content.

Salt. Women with menstrual cramps should carefully avoid excessive salt intake. Too much dietary salt can worsen bloating and fluid retention, thereby contributing to the symptoms of congestive dysmenorrhea. Too much salt intake can also increase high blood pressure and is a risk factor in the development of osteoporosis in menopausal women. Unfortunately, most processed food contains large amounts of salt. Frozen and canned foods are often loaded with salt. In fact, one frozen-food entree can contribute as much as one-half teaspoon of salt to your daily intake.

Large amounts of salt are commonly found in the American diet as table salt (sodium chloride), MSG (monosodium glutamate), and a variety of food additives. Fast foods such as hamburgers, hot dogs, french fries, pizza, and tacos are loaded with salt and saturated fats. Common processed foods such as soups, potato chips, cheese, olives, salad dressings, and catsup (to name only a few) are also loaded with salt. And if this were not bad enough, many people use too much salt in their cooking and seasoning.

For women of all ages, I recommend eliminating added salt in your meals. For flavor, use seasonings such as garlic, herbs, spices, and lemon juice. Avoid processed foods that are high in salt, such as canned foods, olives, pickles, potato chips, tortilla chips, catsup, and salad dressings. Learn to read labels and look for the word sodium (salt). If it appears high on the list of ingredients, don't buy the product. Many brands in the health food stores contain foods labeled "no salt added." Some supermarkets also contain "no added salt" foods in their diet or health food section.

Alcohol. Women with menstrual cramps should avoid alcohol entirely or consume it only in small amounts. Alcohol depletes the body's B-complex vitamins and minerals such as magnesium by disrupting carbohydrate metabolism. Because minerals are important in regulating muscle tension, an alcohol-based nutritional deficiency can worsen muscle spasms at the time of menstruation. Depletion of magnesium and B-complex vitamins can also intensify menstrual fatigue and mood swings.

Alcohol is toxic to the liver and can affect the liver's ability to metabolize hormones efficiently. Excessive alcohol intake has been associated with lack of ovulation and elevated estrogen levels, which can trigger fibroid growth in susceptible women, thereby worsening menstrual pain. It can also trigger heavy menstrual flow, particularly in women who are transitioning into menopause and have a progesterone deficiency. In women with menstrual cramps, excessive estrogen can worsen the congestive symptoms. Estrogen causes fluid and salt retention in the body. When levels are too high, the body can retain excessive amounts of fluid during the premenstrual and menstrual phases of the month.

When used carefully—not exceeding 4 ounces of wine per day, 10 ounces of beer, or 1 ounce of hard liquor—alcohol can have a delightfully relaxing effect. It makes us more sociable and enhances the taste of food. For optimal health, however, I recommend using alcohol only as an occasional treat, not more than once or twice a week. Women who are particularly susceptible to the negative effects of alcohol shouldn't drink at all.

If you entertain often and enjoy social drinking, I recommend that you try nonalcoholic beverages. A nonalcoholic cocktail such as mineral water with a twist of lime or lemon or a dash of bitters is a good substitute. Light wine and beer in small amounts have a lower alcohol content than hard liquor, liqueurs, and regular wine.

Sugar. Like alcohol, sugar depletes the body's B-complex vitamins and minerals, which can worsen muscle tension and irritability as well as nervous tension and anxiety. Unfortunately, sugar addiction is very common in our society among people of all ages. Many people use sweet foods as a way to deal with their frustrations and other upsets. As a result, most Americans eat too much sugar—the average American eats 120 pounds per year.

Many convenience foods, such as bottled salad dressing, ketchup and relish, contain high levels of both sugar and salt. Sugar is the main ingredient in soft drinks and in desserts such as candies, cookies, cakes, and ice cream. Highly sugared foods also promote tooth loss through tooth decay and gum disease. Of even greater significance is the fact that excessive sugar intake can worsen diabetes and blood sugar imbalances.

Try to satisfy your sweet tooth instead with healthier foods such as fruit or grain-based desserts, like oatmeal cookies made with fruit or honey. You will find that small amounts of these foods can satisfy your cravings. Instead of disrupting your mood and energy level, they actually have a healthful and balancing effect.

Caffeine. Coffee, black tea, soft drinks, and chocolate all contain caffeine, a stimulant that many women use to increase their energy level and alertness and decrease fatigue. Caffeine is even used in many over-the-counter menstrual remedies because it does relax blood vessels and promote circulation in the extremities (at the expense of the brain's blood supply). Unfortunately, caffeine has many negative effects on the body. For example, caffeine used in excess increases anxiety, irritability, and mood swings. This can be a real problem for women with anemia who have few emotional and physical reserves.

Caffeine depletes the body's stores of B-complex vitamins and essential minerals, so long-term use can actually increase cramps and menstrual fatigue. Depletion of nutrients like the B-complex vitamins also interferes with carbohydrate metabolism and healthy liver function, which helps to regulate estrogen levels and bleeding. Many menopausal women also complain that caffeine increases the frequency of hot flashes. Coffee, black tea, chocolate, and soft drinks all act to inhibit iron absorption, thus worsening anemia.

How to Substitute Healthy Ingredients in Recipes

Learning how to make substitutions for high-stress ingredients in recipes allows you to use your favorite recipes without compromising your health and well-being. Many recipes start out with ingredients that women with cramps need to avoid, such as dairy products, salt, sugar, chocolate, alcohol and wheat. By eliminating the high-stress foods and replacing them with healthier ingredients, you can still make almost any recipe that you choose. For years I have recommended this method to my patients, who have found that they can still have their favorite dishes, but in a much healthier version.

Some women choose to totally eliminate the high-stress ingredients from a recipe. For example, you can make a pasta and tomato sauce but eliminate the Parmesan cheese topping and use soy parmesan as a substitute, or a Greek salad without the feta cheese. Some of my patients even make pizza without cheese, layering tomato sauce and lots of vegetables on a pizza crust. In many cases, the high-stress ingredients are not necessary in order to make foods taste good.

If you want to retain a high-stress ingredient, you can substantially reduce the amount of that ingredient while still retaining the flavor and taste. Most of us have palates jaded by too much salt, fat, sugar, and other flavorings. In many dishes, all we taste are the additives; we never really enjoy the delicious flavor of the foods themselves. During the years that I have cooked by substituting low-stress ingredients, I have come to enjoy the subtle taste of the dishes much more. Also, I find that my health and vitality continue to improve with the deletion of high-stress ingredients from my food. Use the following information on how to substitute healthy ingredients in your own recipes. The substitutions are easy and simple to make, and should benefit your health greatly.

How to Substitute for Dairy Products

Decrease the amount of milk and dairy-based cheese you use in food preparation and cooking. If you must use cow's cheese in cooking, decrease the amount by one-half to two-thirds so that it becomes a flavoring or garnish rather than a major source of fat and protein. You can add soft tofu to recipes to replace cheese. I have done this often with lasagna by layering the noodles with tofu and topping with melted soy cheese for a delicious dish. The tofu, which is bland, takes on the taste of the tomato sauce. If you cannot give up milk products, try to use the lower-fat cheeses now available. Goat's or sheep's cheese in small amounts can also replace cow's cheese because the fat they contain is more easily emulsified in the body.

Use soy, vegan and rice cheese made without casein in food preparation and cooking. Soy cheese is an excellent substitute for dairy-based cheese. It is lower in fat and salt, and the fat it contains isn't saturated. The health food stores offer many brands that come in many different flavors, such as mozzarella, cheddar, American, and jack. The quality of these products keeps improving all the time. You can use soy cheese as a perfect cheese substitute in sandwiches, salads, pizzas, lasagnas, and casseroles. Vegan and rice cheeses are very good substitutes for dairy cheese, also.

Replace milk in recipes. For cow's milk, substitute rice, almond, coconut, flaxseed, hempseed, sunflower seed and soy milk. These non-dairy milks are readily available in health food stores and many supermarkets. Many nondairy milks are good sources of calcium and can be used for drinking, eating, or baking.

Substitute flax oil for butter. Flax oil is the best substitute for butter that I have found. It is a golden, rich oil that looks and tastes quite a bit like butter. It is delicious used on anything on which you'd normally use butter—toast, rice, popcorn, steamed vegetables, and potatoes. It is extremely high in essential fatty acids—the type of fat that is very healthy for a woman's body. Essential fatty acids help to promote normal hormonal function. Flax oil is quite perishable, however, since it is sensitive to heat and light. You can't cook with it—the food must be cooked first, and then the flax oil can be added before serving. It also must be refrigerated. I highly recommend using flax oil because of its many health benefits. You can find it in health food stores. Ground flaxseeds are excellent used in shakes, smoothies or stirred into hot cereal and can also be purchased in health food stores or online. It has the same anti-inflammatory benefits as flax oil.

How to Substitute for Caffeinated Foods and Beverages

Use coffee and tea substitutes. For drinking, the best coffee substitutes are the grain-based beverages like Postum and Cafix. Some women may find that discontinuing coffee abruptly is too difficult because of withdrawal symptoms such as headaches. If this is a concern for you, decrease your total coffee intake gradually to one-half to one cup per day. Use coffee substitutes the rest of the time. This will help prevent withdrawal symptoms.

Use decaffeinated coffee or tea as a transition beverage. If you cannot give up coffee immediately, you can start substituting water-process decaffeinated coffee for the real thing. Then try to wean yourself from coffee altogether.

Use herbal teas for energy and vitality. Many women drink coffee for the pick-up they get from it. Those morning cups of coffee allow them to wake up and function through the day. Use ginger instead. It is a great herbal stimulant that won't wreck your health. To make ginger tea, grate a few teaspoons of fresh ginger root into a pot of hot water. Boil and steep. Serve with honey. Green tea is also a great, healthful tea with only a small amount of caffeine. It can be used safely except by women who suffer from anxiety and panic attacks and are very sensitive to the effects of caffeine.

Avoid caffeinated soft drinks. Instead try a glass of sparkling water with a slice of lemon or lime and a dash of bitters. This is a great festive drink to enjoy at home or even at social events and get-togethers.

How to Substitute for Chocolate

Substitute carob for chocolate. Unsweetened carob tastes like chocolate but is far more nutritious. It is a member of the legume family and is high in calcium. You can purchase carob in chunk form as a substitute for chocolate candy or as a powder to be used in baking or drinks. Be careful, however, not to overindulge.

Carob, like chocolate, is high in calories and fat. It should be considered a treat and cooking aid to be used only in small amounts.

Caffeine Content of Beverages and Foods

(listed in order of caffeine content)

Product	Caffeine per Serving
Coffee (per cup)	
Drip (average)	146 mg
Percolated (average)	110 mg
Coffee—instant (per cup)	
Folgers	97.5 mg
Maxwell House	94 mg
Nescafe	81 mg
Decaffeinated Coffee (per cup)	
Taster's Choice	3.5 mg
Tea (per cup)	
Tetley	63.5 mg
Lipton	52 mg
Constant Comment	29 mg
Green Tea	24-40 mg
Soft Drinks (per 12 oz. can)	
Mountain Dew	55 mg
Diet Dr. Pepper	54 mg
Coke Classic	46 mg
Diet Coke	46 mg
Pepsi	38.4 mg
Diet Pepsi	36 mg
Hot Chocolate Drinks (per cup)	
Cocoa	13 mg
Candy (per oz.)	
Ghirardelli Dark Chocolate	24 mg
Hershey's Milk Chocolate	4 mg

How to Substitute for Sugar

Cut the amount of sweetener in your recipes by one-third to one-half. Americans tend to eat too much sugar. That is a fact based simply on our tendency to consume close to 120 pounds of sugar a year per person. Most of us grew up on highly sugared soft drinks, candy, and rich pastries—no wonder the incidence of diabetes is soaring among our population. I have found that as women decrease their sugar intake, most begin to really enjoy the subtle flavors of the foods they eat.

Substitute xylitol and stevia for sugar. Xylitol has been used instead of sugar for cooking and recipes. It has one third the calories of sugar and has health benefits for your teeth and gums. It is one of my favorite sugar substitutes. Stevia is another excellent sweetener for teas and other beverages and has no calories.

Substitute concentrated sweeteners. Concentrated sweeteners such as honey and maple syrup have a sweeter taste per quantity used than table sugar. This will allow you to cut down on the actual amount of sugar in a recipe. If you use a concentrated sweetener in place of sugar in an ordinary recipe, reduce the liquid content in the recipe by ¼ cup. If no liquid is used in the recipe, add 3 to 5 tablespoons of flour for each ¾ cup of concentrated sweetener to ensure the proper texture.

Substitute fruit for sugar in pastries. In making muffins and cookies, you may want to try eliminating sugar altogether and adding extra fruits like bananas and applesauce and nuts.

How to Substitute for Salt

Substitute potassium-based products for table salt (sodium chloride). Potassium-based products such as Morton's Salt Substitute are much healthier and will not aggravate heart disease or hypertension.

Substitute powdered seaweeds such as kelp or nori to season vegetables, grains, and salads. They are high in essential iodine and trace elements.

Use herbs instead of salt for flavoring. Their flavors are much more subtle and will help even the most jaded palate appreciate the taste of fresh fruits, vegetables, and meats.

Use low-sodium content liquid flavoring agents. Low-salt soy sauce and Bragg's Amino Acids, a liquid soybean-based flavoring agent, are delicious when used in cooking as salt substitutes. When you add them to soups, casseroles, stir-fries, and other dishes at the end of the cooking process, you will find that you need only a small amount for intense flavoring.

How to Substitute for Wheat Flour

While consuming whole grains has many health benefits, some women with menstrual cramps and other women's health issues like fibroid tumors may find that they are allergic to or intolerant of wheat. Most women are surprised by this discovery, since wheat is one of the staples of our culture and is eaten by most people at almost every meal. However, wheat contains a protein called gluten, which is highly allergenic and difficult for the body to break down, absorb, and assimilate. Women with wheat intolerance are prone to fatigue, depression, sinusitis, allergies, bloating, intestinal gas, and bowel changes.

In my clinical experience, when women are nutritionally sensitive, wheat consumption can often worsen emotional symptoms and lower energy levels. I have observed how wheat (along with other foods) can trigger emotional symptoms, bloating and fatigue in PMS patients, especially during the week or two before the onset of menses. Many menopausal women tolerate wheat poorly because their digestive tracts are beginning to show the wear and tear of aging and don't produce enough enzymes to break down wheat easily.

Women with allergies often find that wheat intensifies nasal and sinus congestion, as well as fatigue. I also find that women with poor resistance and a tendency toward infections may need to eliminate wheat from their diets to boost their immune systems. Since wheat is leavened with yeast, it should also be avoided by women with candida.

Use gluten-free grains. If you suffer from any of these conditions, as well as dull aching, cramping and bloating with PMS, you should probably eliminate wheat from your diet. I have found over the years that the least stressful grain for women with menstrual cramping, pain and bloating are grains like brown rice, millet, quinoa, wild rice, amaranth and buckwheat. For example, buckwheat is not commonly eaten in our culture, so most women never develop an intolerance to it. Also, it is not in the same plant family as wheat and other grains. Buckwheat is actually the fruit-like structure of the plant rather than a grass. Other grains such as wild rice, quinoa, and amaranth should be tried as well. These are available in health food stores in pastas and cereals.

I recommend that you and use the many gluten-free breads, breakfast cereals, bagels, English muffins, cookies, pasta and other flour based foods that are readily available in health food stores and many supermarkets. Oats and rye, which also contain gluten, should be eliminated along with wheat if your symptoms are moderate to severe. Gluten-free oats, however, are available in health food stores and some supermarkets.

How to Substitute for Alcohol

Alcohol depletes the body's vitamin B and minerals, disrupts carbohydrate metabolism, and intensifies symptoms of PMS related cramping and bloating. Alcohol is toxic to the liver and can disrupt the liver's ability to metabolize hormones, thus causing higher-than-normal estrogen.

Use low-alcohol or nonalcoholic products for cooking. Substitute low-alcohol or nonalcoholic wine or beer when cooking or preparing sauces and marinades. You will retain much of the flavor that alcohol imparts and you'll decrease the stress factor substantially.

If you want a festive drink to enjoy at social events and get-togethers with family and friends, try a glass of sparkling water with a slice of lemon or lime and a dash of bitters. It is a very refreshing and fun nonalcoholic beverage.

Substitutes for Common High-Stress Ingredients

3/4 cup sugar	3/4 cup xylitol 1/2 cup honey 1/4 cup molasses 1/2 cup maple syrup 1/2 ounce barley malt 1 cup apple butter 2 cups apple juice
1 cup milk	1 cup soy, rice, nut, or grain milk
1 tablespoon butter	1 tablespoon flax oil (must be used raw and unheated)
1/2 teaspoon salt	1 tablespoon miso 1/2 teaspoon potassium chloride salt substitute 1/2 teaspoon Mrs. Dash, Spike 1/2 teaspoon herbs (basil, tarragon, oregano, etc.)
1 1/2 cups cocoa	1 cup powdered carob
1 square chocolate	3/4 tablespoon powdered carob
1 tablespoon coffee	1 tablespoon decaffeinated coffee 1 tablespoon Postum, Cafix, or other grain-based coffee substitute
4 ounces wine	4 ounces light wine
8 ounces beer	8 ounces near beer
1 cup white flour	1 cup barley flour (pie crust) 1 cup rice flour (cookies, cakes, breads)

Healthy Food Shopping List

Vegetables

Beets	Eggplant	Radicchio
Bok choy	Garlic	Radishes
Broccoli	Green beans	Rutabagas
Brussels sprouts	Horseradish	Sauerkraut
Cabbage	Kale	Spinach
Carrots	Lettuce	Squash
Cauliflower	Mustard greens	Sweet Potatoes
Celery	Okra	Tomatoes
Chard	Onions	Turnips
Cilantro	Parsley	Turnip Greens
Collard	Parsnips	Watercress
Cucumbers	Peas (all varieties)	Yams
Dandelion greens	Potatoes	

Legumes	**Whole Grains**	**Seeds and Nuts**
Adzuki	Amaranth	Almonds
Black	Barley	Cashews
Black-eyed peas	Brown rice	Filberts
Cannellini	Buckwheat	Flaxseeds
Fava	Corn	Macadamia
Garbanzo	Millet	Pecan
Kidney	Oatmeal	Pumpkin seeds
Lentils	Quinoa	Sesame seeds
Navy	Rye	Sunflower seeds
Red		Walnuts
Soy: tofu, tempeh		
Turtle beans		

Healthy Food Shopping List (continued)

Fruits
Acai berries
Apples
Avocado
Bananas
Berries
Blueberries
Raspberries
Strawberries
Coconuts
Goji berries
Kiwi
Noni
Olives
Pomegranates
Pears
Seasonal Fruits

Sweeteners
Brown rice syrup
Honey
Maple syrup
Molasses
Stevia
Xylitol

Beverages
Coconut water
Grain based coffee
Substitute
Herbal tea
Green tea
Water

Meats
Fish
Free-range poultry
Game meat
Organic lean red meat
Seafood (in
moderation)

Oils
Flax
Macadamia
Olive
Safflower
Sesame
Walnut

Foods from Other Cultures
Gomasio
Jicama
Miso
Seaweed (like kelp,
dulse, nori, wakane)
Tamari soy sauce
Umeboshi plums

Dairy Substitutes
Hemp milk
Nut milk
Rice milk
Soy milk
Soy, coconut, almond,
rice or hemp cheeses,
cream cheese, yogurt,
and frozen desserts
*Avoid all soy products
containing
hydrogenated oil.

Herbs & Spices
Basil
Black pepper
Cayenne pepper
Chamomile
Chili pepper, dried
Cilantro
Cinnamon, ground
Cloves
Coriander
Cumin
Dill
Ginger
Licorice
Mustard seeds
Oregano
Peppermint
Poppy
Rosemary
Sage
Tarragon
Thyme
Turmeric

5

Menus, Meal Plans & Recipes

This is one of my favorite chapters because it addresses the pleasure and enjoyment that women can have when preparing and eating health-enhancing foods. My personal interest in meal planning goes back to my medical training years when I first saw the dramatic benefits that a low-stress, high-nutrient diet had on my own menstrual cramps and symptoms. My health problems cleared up beautifully when I made the necessary nutritional changes. Over the years, I have seen that good nutritional habits have equally beneficial effects on my patients' health problems. Many of my patients have a dramatic reduction in menstrual cramps and congestive symptoms in a very short period of time when they eliminate high-stress foods.

Many patients have asked me for specific menus, recipes and meal plans, to help them implement their own self-care program. Most cookbooks contain recipes that are too high in the nutrients that can worsen cramps, such as animal fats, dairy products, caffeine, sugar, and salt. More nutrition-conscious cookbooks present low calorie, "light dishes" that eliminate the high-stress ingredients, but still don't give women with menstrual cramps the therapeutic levels of specific nutrients they need. As a result, I've developed these resources for many of my patients to assist them in their healing.

This chapter contains many menus and recipes that have provided very beneficial therapeutic results for my patients. One very important observation I've made in working with thousands of patients is that there is no one size fits all diet. Women have very differing dietary and nutritional needs.

For example, some women feel their best on a high carbohydrate, vegetarian emphasis diet while other women need a more meat-based high protein diet. Both of these types of diets can successfully help to eliminate menstrual cramps, as long as they are high in essential nutrients and eliminate foods that trigger pain and cramping symptoms. As a result, I have included menus, meal plans and recipes in this book that provide you with both of these dietary options to fit your specific needs!

I am also aware of the busy lives that many women lead and the time demands that so many of us face; thus many of the recipes are quick, simple, and easy to prepare. Best of all, these recipes are delicious as well as healthy. I hope that you find trying these new dishes to be a delightful adventure as well as beneficial for your health.

Breakfast Menus

These delicious breakfast menus have been developed to help reduce and prevent symptoms of menstrual cramps. All the dishes contain high levels of the essential nutrients that women with menstrual cramps need. The recipes use no high-stress ingredients, yet they will create tasty and nutritious breakfast dishes that you can enjoy you can also use these as idea generators for your own meal planning.

Breakfast has been one of the easiest meals for my patients to restructure along healthier lines. It tends to be a smaller and simpler meal. You may want to make healthful dietary changes in your breakfast first and then move on to lunch and dinner.

Flax shake with protein powder
and fresh fruit
~~~~~~~~~~~~~~

Blueberry and spirulina smoothie
~~~~~~~~~~~~~~

Millet cereal with raisins and
cinnamon
Nondairy yogurt
Chamomile tea
~~~~~~~~~~~~~~

Rice and flaxseed pancakes
Banana
Vanilla nondairy milk
~~~~~~~~~~~~~~

Oatmeal with raspberries
Chamomile tea
~~~~~~~~~~~~~~

Nondairy yogurt with granola
and ground flaxseed
Peppermint tea
~~~~~~~~~~~~~~

Scrambled eggs with turkey
bacon
Ginger tea
Orange slices
~~~~~~~~~~~~~~

Omelette with chicken sausage
Roasted grain beverage (coffee
substitute)
Apple slices
~~~~~~~~~~~~~~

Lunch and Dinner Menus

Here is a variety of delicious menus you can choose from when planning your meals. You can use these menu plans or as idea generators to fit your own taste and needs. These dishes contain many nutritious and healthful ingredients for menstrual cramps relief.

Use these menus as helpful guidelines throughout the entire month. Your nutritional status on a day-by-day basis determines in part how likely you are to have menstrual cramp and pain symptoms. These dishes should help to diminish the severity of your symptoms because they eliminate high-stress ingredients.

Soup Meals
Split pea soup
Corn muffins
Fresh applesauce
~~~~~~~~~~~~~~~

Chicken and wild rice soup
Cole slaw
Millet bread with flax oil
~~~~~~~~~~~~~~~

Vegetable soup with brown rice
Steamed kale
Baked potato with flax oil
Apple slices
~~~~~~~~~~~~~~~

Lentil soup
Herbed brown rice
Broccoli with lemon
~~~~~~~~~~~~~~~

Tomato soup
Potato salad with low-fat mayonnaise
Celery and carrot sticks
~~~~~~~~~~~~~~~

Salad Meals
Spinach salad with turkey bacon or tofu
Corn muffins with flax oil
Orange slices
~~~~~~~~~~~~~~~

Beet salad with goat cheese
Rice crackers with fresh fruit preserves
~~~~~~~~~~~~~~~

Romaine salad with grilled salmon
Gluten-free bread and olive oil dip
~~~~~~~~~~~~~~~

Low-fat potato salad
Cole slaw
Hard boiled eggs
Melon slices
~~~~~~~~~~~~~~~

Meat Meals

Poached salmon with lemon
Herbed brown rice
Steamed carrots with honey

~~~~~~~~~~~~~~

Roasted chicken with herbs
Baked potato with flax oil
Broccoli with lemon

~~~~~~~~~~~~~~

Broiled trout with dill
Mixed green salad with vinaigrette
Green peas and onions
Apple slices

~~~~~~~~~~~~~~

Grilled shrimp with olive oil and
lemon
Wild rice
Steamed kale

~~~~~~~~~~~~~~

One-Dish Vegetable Meals

Vegetarian tacos with black beans,
brown rice, avocados and low-salt
salsa

~~~~~~~~~~~~~~

Stir-fry with mixed vegetables,
brown rice and tofu
Orange slices

~~~~~~~~~~~~~~

Pasta with tomato sauce, broccoli,
carrots, olive oil and garlic
Green salad with vinaigrette

~~~~~~~~~~~~~~

Hummus dip
Eggplant dip (babaganoush)
Mixed raw vegetable slices
including carrots, red bell peppers,
and radishes

~~~~~~~~~~~~~~

Brown rice and almond tabouli
Mixed olives
Melon slices

~~~~~~~~~~~~~~

Breakfast Recipes

 Beverages

These drinks are designed to be delicious, nutritious, and to help you heal from menstrual cramps. They include therapeutic herbal teas, power smoothies that are rich in fruits, raw seeds, nuts, protein powder, green foods and nondairy milk. These ingredients are all recommended for preventing and treating your symptoms.

These wonderful drinks contain high levels of essential nutrients that help regulate your hormonal balance and relax pain and tension in the muscles of the pelvis and lower extremities. You can enjoy these beverages throughout the month, and not just during your symptom time, as their high mineral and other nutrient content is beneficial for the entire body.

Relaxant Herb Tea   **Serves 2**

2 cups water
1 teaspoon chamomile leaves
1 teaspoon peppermint leaves
1 teaspoon honey (if desired)

Bring the water to a boil. Place herbs in water and stir. Turn heat to low and simmer for 15 minutes.

Peppermint and chamomile are both muscle relaxants and antispasmodic herbs, so they can provide relief of menstrual pain and cramping. They also help calm the mood.

Ginger Tea **Serves 4**

Ginger makes a warming, delicious tea and is beneficial to your circulation. It is also a powerful anti-inflammatory herb. If the tea is too strong add more water.

5 cups water
3 tablespoons ginger coarsely chopped
½ lemon (optional)
Honey (or other sweetener, to taste)

Add ginger to the water in a cooking pot. Bring to a boil and then turn heat to low. Steep for 15 or 20 minutes. Squeeze lemon into tea and serve with honey or your favorite sweetener.

Heavenly Strawberry Coconut Smoothie **Serves 2**

This drink fits its name! It is absolutely scrumptious as well as good for you. If you don't have a high-speed blender and you are using whole raw cashews I recommend that you chop them up beforehand. Otherwise raw cashew butter is a good substitute.

1 cup coconut drink, unsweetened (Coconut Dream brand preferred)
1 cup strawberries – fresh or frozen
1 tablespoon raw coconut flour
2 tablespoons raw cashews (10-15)
1 banana, sliced

Combine all ingredients in a blender. Puree until smooth and serve.

Peachy Flax Smoothie   **Serves 2**

½ cup orange juice
½ cup unsweetened rice milk
1 cup peaches – fresh or frozen
1 tablespoon rice protein powder
2 teaspoons ground flaxseed
1 banana, sliced

Combine all ingredients in a blender. Puree until smooth and serve.

If using frozen peaches, chopping the peaches beforehand will reduce the puree time in the blender.

Individuals who have weak liver function in addition to diminished enzyme production may not be able to tolerate seeds, nuts, and their oils. The amount of seeds and nuts in the previous recipes may be reduced or eliminated entirely.

Flaxseed oil is actually beneficial for liver function but may be halved in quantity or even eliminated from the above recipes for people who have severely impaired liver function. The amount of flaxseed oil used in these recipes may then be gradually increased as liver function improves.

Blueberry and Greens Shake   **Serves 2**

This drink is a powerhouse of nutrients! The chlorella and spirulina are highly beneficial green foods. They are rich in nutrients like beta-carotene and help to detoxify the liver. They are readily available at health food stores.

1 cup nondairy milk
⅔ cup blueberries – fresh or frozen
2 tablespoons protein powder
½ teaspoon chlorella
½ teaspoon spirulina
Sprinkle of Truvia (optional)

In a blender puree the nondairy milk and blueberries. Add rest of ingredients and blend well.

Delicious Green Drink   **Serves 1**

½ cup Concord grape juice
¼ cup water
1 tablespoon ground flaxseed
½ teaspoon chlorella powder
½ teaspoon spirulina powder

Mix all ingredients together in a glass or puree in a blender.

Simple Flax Smoothie   **Serves 2**

Flaxseed is not only a tasty addition to smoothies but it is also very nutritious. Flaxseed is high in essential fatty acids, calcium, magnesium, and potassium.

1 cup vanilla nondairy milk
2 tablespoons ground flaxseed
1 banana

Combine all ingredients in a blender. Blend until smooth and serve.

Healthy, Quick Breakfasts

I love breakfast and it is the most important meal to start your day off right. Unfortunately, most American breakfasts include wheat and dairy products, such as yogurt, wheat toast, wheat and sugary cereals with milk, sweet rolls and white flour pancakes and waffles. As I explained in Chapter 4, dairy products and wheat can worsen the symptoms of menstrual cramps and PMS (which often occurs concurrently).

I have included in this section many recipes to start your day healthfully. The recipes include both whole grain, carbohydrate based entrees as well as protein-rich dishes, depending on the type of diet that makes you feel your best. Both types of dishes, however, will benefit menstrual cramp symptoms by eliminating wheat, dairy, caffeine and sugar at breakfast.

The whole grain dishes are rich in ground flaxseed, soy, and gluten-free grains, all of which can be useful in reducing your symptoms. Gluten containing grains have been eliminated because the protein found in wheat can trigger symptoms of bloating, digestive disturbances, and fatigue. The protein-based entrees have been created using eggs and healthy breakfast meats.

Quinoa Cereal with Strawberries   **Serves 2**

1 ½ cups cooked quinoa
1 cup nondairy milk
½ cup strawberries
2 teaspoons honey or other sweetener

Combine quinoa and nondairy milk in a saucepan. Simmer for 5 minutes. Stir in honey and garnish with raspberries.

Quinoa with Prunes **Serves 2**

This is one of my all-time favorite hot cereals. The plums are delicious and add a nice texture. Quinoa is a small, protein rich grain. When cooked the grains are small and fluffy. I recommend making a pot of quinoa the night before.

1 ½ cups cooked quinoa
1 cup nondairy milk
4-6 dried prunes, chopped
2 tablespoons flaxseed oil
2 teaspoons xylitol, honey, or maple syrup (if using unsweetened milk)
Pinch of salt (optional)

In a saucepan combine quinoa, nondairy milk, salt, and dried plums. Heat thoroughly and simmer on low heat for 5-10 minutes until plums have softened. Serve with flaxseed oil and sweetener.

Maple Cinnamon Oatmeal **Serves 2**

1 cup gluten-free quick oats
1 ¾ cups water
1-2 tablespoons flaxseed oil
2 teaspoons maple syrup
Pinch of cinnamon (to taste)
Pinch of salt

Boil water in a saucepan. Add gluten-free oats and reduce to medium heat. Cook for one minute and stir. Cover, and remove oatmeal from heat. Serve in 2-3 minutes.

Stir in maple syrup, flaxseed oil, cinnamon and salt.

Strawberries and Cream Oatmeal   **Serves 2**

1 cup gluten-free quick oats
½ cup strawberries, chopped
½ nondairy milk
1 ¼ cups water
1-2 tablespoons flaxseed oil
2 teaspoons honey or stevia
Pinch of salt (optional)

Bring water and nondairy milk to a boil in a saucepan. Add gluten-free oats and reduce to medium heat. Cook for one minute and stir. Cover, and remove oatmeal from heat. Serve in 2-3 minutes. Stir in sweetener, flaxseed oil, salt and top with strawberries.

Banana Nut Muffins   **Makes 14-18**

These moist muffins are a twist on the classic recipe using cashews instead of walnuts. Very tasty!

1½ cups rice flour
1 teaspoon baking powder
½ teaspoon baking soda
3 ripe bananas, mashed
¼ teaspoon cinnamon
6 packets of Truvia (¼ cup)
¼ cup honey
¼ cup safflower oil
⅓ cup cashews, chopped

Preheat oven to 350 degrees. Mix all dry ingredients and wet ingredients separately. Combine and mix well. Fill muffin cups ⅔ with the batter.

Pumpkin Muffins **Makes 14-18 muffins**

1½ cups rice flour
½ teaspoon baking powder
½ teaspoon baking soda
1 cup pumpkin
1 teaspoon cinnamon
¼ teaspoon nutmeg
¼ cup chopped almonds (optional)
3 tablespoons molasses
3 tablespoons safflower oil
½ cup raisins
2 eggs
½ cup nondairy milk
1 teaspoon vanilla extract
Pinch of salt

Preheat oven to 400 degrees. Line a muffin tin with paper muffin cups.

Combine all dry ingredients and mix thoroughly. In a separate bowl beat the two eggs and then combine the remainder of the wet ingredients. Add the wet ingredients to the dry and mix thoroughly.

Fill muffin cups ⅔ with the batter. Cook for 18-20 minutes or until thoroughly cooked.

Flaxseed Pancakes   **Makes 8 pancakes (serves 2-4)**

Xylitol is an excellent sugar substitute for cooking and baking that can be found at most health food stores. Xylitol is easy to use because it has a 1:1 ratio with sugar. Yet, this product has 40% fewer calories than sugar and is beneficial for your teeth and gums.

1 cup gluten-free flour
1 cup unsweetened rice milk
1 egg
2 tablespoons xylitol
1 tablespoon ground flaxseed
1 teaspoon baking powder
½ teaspoon baking soda
¼ teaspoon salt
3 tablespoons almond oil, keeping 1 tbsp. for cooking
Maple syrup (optional)
Fruit jam (optional)

Mix the dry and wet ingredients in separate bowls. Combine all the ingredients and mix thoroughly. Cook on medium heat and use a small amount of oil to grease the pan if needed. When pancakes bubble in the center flip and cook for 1-2 minutes until cooked thoroughly. Serve with maple syrup or all-fruit jam. Delicious!

Egg and Sausage Scramble   **Serves 2**

4 eggs
4 turkey breakfast sausages
2 slice of gluten-free toast
Salt and pepper (optional)
2 teaspoons olive oil
Serve with ½ cup applesauce

Warm a frying pan on medium heat and add olive oil. Beat egg gently in a small bowl and set aside. Chop the sausages into small pieces - this will help them to cook faster. Add sausages to the pan and cook for several minutes until sausages are brown. Turn heat to low and add eggs to the pan and scramble with the sausage. Add a pinch of salt and pepper. Serve with toast and applesauce.

Bake for 20-25 minutes until cooked through.

Mushroom Onion Scramble   **Serves 2**

The mushrooms and onion give this egg scramble a great texture. The water helps make the eggs fluffier.

4 eggs
1 tablespoon water
¼ onion
2-3 mushrooms
1 tablespoon olive oil
Salt and pepper (optional)

Dice the mushrooms and onion. Next, beat the 4 eggs together with 1 tablespoon water. Preheat the frying pan on medium heat and add 1 tablespoon olive oil. Add onion and mushroom and cook for about 3 minutes until onions are translucent and add eggs. Let sit for about 30 second and then start to scramble with your spatula. Add a pinch of salt and pepper and serve.

Spinach and Tomato Scramble   **Serves 2**

The Parmesan cheese adds a delightful saltiness and tang to this dish.

4 eggs, beaten
1 tablespoon water
2 tablespoons diced onion
¼ tomato, chopped
12 spinach leaves, chopped
1 tablespoon olive oil
Salt and pepper (optional)
Parmesan cheese - or soy Parmesan (optional)

Beat the 4 eggs together with 1 tablespoon water. Preheat the frying pan on medium heat and add 1 tablespoon olive oil. Add onion and cook for about 3 minutes until onions are translucent. Next add eggs, spinach and tomato. Let sit for about 15 seconds and then start to scramble with your spatula. Sprinkle on a small amount of Parmesan cheese, add a pinch of salt and pepper and serve.

Spreads and Sauces

These spreads and sauces contain highly concentrated levels of ingredients that help to relax menstrual cramp-related pain and muscle tension and help to relieve congestion. Serve with rice cakes, crackers, corn bread, or even spread on a banana for a delicious treat.

Fresh Applesauce   **Serves 2**

2 ½ apples
½ cup fresh apple juice
½ teaspoon cinnamon
½ teaspoon ginger

Peel apples and cut into quarters; remove cores. Combine all ingredients in a food processor. Blend until smooth.

Sesame-Tofu Spread   **Serves 4**

¼ cup soft tofu
¼ cup raw sesame butter
¼ cup honey

Combine all ingredients in a blender. Serve with rice cakes or crackers.

Lunch and Dinner Recipes

These high-nutrient, scrumptious lunch and dinner dishes are designed to help prevent and relieve your symptoms. The ingredients do not include red meat, dairy products, or wheat, all of which can worsen your symptoms. Mix and match these dishes as you please. You might combine soups and salads or whole grains, legumes and vegetables for a complete vegetarian emphasis or meat-based meal, depending on your needs for carbohydrates and protein.

The main course dishes are all extremely healthful for women with menstrual cramps and pain. You can enjoy these dishes particularly during the second half of your menstrual cycle when your symptoms are worse, but for optimal health and well-being, I recommend their use all month long.

 Soups

Split Pea Soup   Serves 4

¾ cup split peas
5 cups low-sodium chicken broth
⅔ cup carrot, chopped
¾ cup onion, diced
Tamari soy sauce – to taste (optional)

Bring the water to a boil and add the split peas, onion, carrots, and chicken broth. Reduce heat to low and simmer for 50 minutes – 1 hour, stirring occasionally. If water begins to cook off add up to an extra cup of water. Add a dash of tamari soy sauce for a saltier flavor.

Black Bean Soup   Serves 4

This recipe is easy and makes a delicious, filling soup.

1 can black beans (14 ounce), rinsed
5 cups low-sodium vegetable broth
1 cup onion, diced
⅔ cup carrot, chopped
⅔ cup red pepper, chopped
¼ teaspoon cumin
Tamari soy sauce – to taste (optional)

Bring the water to a boil and add all ingredients. Reduce heat to low and simmer for 30 minutes, stirring occasionally. If water begins to cook off add up to an extra cup of water. Add a dash of tamari soy sauce for a saltier flavor.

Chicken Rice Soup   Serves 4-6

Few things make me feel better than a bowl of homemade chicken rice soup. I have an easy tip to add extra flavor to your soup: If you used the meat from a roasted, skin-on chicken you can add some of the skin to the soup while it is cooking. This will add depth and richness to your soup. Remove the skin when the soup has finished cooking.

6 cups low-sodium chicken broth
⅔ cup carrot
1 cup celery, diced
1 cup cooked chicken, diced
⅔ cup onion, diced
⅔ cup brown rice, cooked
Tamari soy sauce – to taste (optional)

Bring water to a boil and add all ingredients. Reduce heat to low and simmer for 30 minutes, stirring occasionally. If water begins to cook off add up to an extra cup of water. Add a dash of tamari soy sauce for a saltier flavor.

Butternut Squash Soup   **Serves 4**

This soup has been a long-time favorite of mine. I adore the light, creamy texture. Adding maple syrup enhances the natural sweetness of the squash.

½ onion, diced
1 cup low-sodium chicken broth
2 cups pureed butternut squash - fresh or frozen (fresh is preferred)
½ teaspoon cinnamon
1½ cups nondairy milk
2 teaspoons maple syrup
1 tablespoon safflower oil
½-¾ teaspoon salt

In a large saucepan heat the oil on medium heat. Add the onion and cook until translucent. Add the butternut squash, chicken broth, cinnamon and salt. Mix well and simmer for 5 minutes. Add nondairy milk and maple syrup. Simmer on low heat for ten minutes. Stir frequently while cooking the soup.

Optional: To make extra creamy, blend the soup when it has finished cooking. Wait for the soup to cool before blending.

Salads

Zingy Watercress Salad   Serves 4

I enjoy the refreshing bitterness of watercress. This salad pairs well with green apple. Watercress has a strong flavor and a little goes a long way.

1 cup watercress, coarsely chopped
4 cups butter lettuce (or other soft lettuce), coarsely chopped
2 teaspoons scallions, finely chopped
½ green apple, chopped
1 ounce goat cheese, crumbled
Vinaigrette dressing

In a large bowl toss the watercress, butter lettuce, green onion, and apple together with the vinaigrette dressing (to taste). On top of the salad crumble the goat cheese.

Caesar Salad   Serves 2-4

I love Caesar salads. They have been my favorite salad for years! The crispy romaine lettuce and creamy dressing is a perfect match. I like to use anchovies because they are delicious in this salad and also full of healthy anti-inflammatory oils. I prefer the filets packed in olive oil.

1 head of romaine lettuce, chopped – about 6 cups
4 tablespoons light Caesar dressing
4 anchovy filets, chopped
⅔ cup gluten-free croutons
1½ tablespoons grated Parmesan cheese
1 cup roast chicken, cubed (optional)

In a large mixing bowl pour Caesar's dressing over lettuce. Mix well so that leaves are evenly coated with dressing. Add croutons, Parmesan cheese, anchovies, and toss well. Top with roasted chicken and serve.

Potato Salad   **Serves 4-6**

This is a light twist on classic potato salad and makes a great side dish. The vegetables add a delightful crunchiness. This salad pairs well with a turkey or chicken sandwich.

10-12 small red potatoes, cut into bite size pieces (about 2 cups)
2 tablespoons diced celery
2 tablespoons diced red onion
2 tablespoons diced red pepper
1 heaping tablespoon diced water chestnuts
1 hardboiled egg, yolk removed
1 heaping tablespoon mayonnaise
1 teaspoon whole grain Dijon mustard

Steam the potatoes for 15-20 minutes or until fork tender and let cool. Chop up all the vegetables into small pieces and set aside. Chop egg white and set aside.

In a mixing bowl add vegetables, mayonnaise and mustard to the potatoes and mix well. Add egg, mix, and serve.

Scrumptious Veggie Salad   **Serves 4-6**

This is one of my favorite salads! It pairs wonderfully with soups and sandwiches.

1 head red lettuce, chopped into bite size pieces
1 large tomato, chopped
2 green onions, sliced
6 mushrooms, sliced
¾ cup kidney beans – canned works well
1 avocado, sliced
¼ cup sunflower seeds
Vinaigrette dressing (to taste)

Combine all ingredients except for avocado in a large salad bowl. Mix in Vinaigrette Dressing and top with avocado slices before serving.

Radicchio and Orange Salad   **Serves 4-6**

This is a sophisticated and delicious salad. I love salads with "extras" such as fruit or a little bit of goat cheese.

6 cups salad greens
½ radicchio, sliced thin
⅓ red onion, sliced very thin
3 ounces goat cheese
1 medium sized orange, peeled and cut into bite size segments
Orange vinaigrette

In a large bowl combine salad greens, radicchio, onion, and oranges. Pour vinaigrette, to taste, over salad and toss. Add goat cheese before serving.

Grains and Starches

Wild Rice   Serves 2

⅔ cup wild rice
2 ½ cups water
½ teaspoon salt

Wash rice with cold water. Combine all ingredients in a cooking pot and bring to a rapid boil. Turn flame to low, cover, and cook without stirring (about 45 minutes) until rice is tender but not mushy. Uncover and fluff with a fork. Cook an additional 5 minutes, and then serve.

Kasha   Serves 4

1 cup kasha (buckwheat groats)
3 ¼ cups water
Pinch of salt

Bring ingredients to a boil, lower heat, and simmer for 25 minutes or until soft. The grains should be fluffy, like rice.

For breakfast, blend in blender with water until creamy. Add almond milk, sesame milk, or sunflower milk, and cinnamon, apple butter, raisins, or berries.

Delicious Baked Sweet Potato   Serves 4

4 sweet potatoes
1 teaspoon olive oil
1 tablespoon flax oil for each potato

Preheat oven to 400° F. Wash the potatoes, then rub with olive oil. Bake for 45 to 60 minutes, or until soft when pierced with a fork. Garnish with flax oil. Honey, maple syrup, or chopped raw pecans may also be used.

Baked Potato   **Serves 4**

4 russet or Idaho potatoes
2 teaspoons olive oil
1 tablespoon flax oil for each potato

Preheat oven to 400° F. Wash the potatoes, rub them with olive oil, and bake for 45 to 60 minutes, or until soft when pierced with a fork. Garnish with flax oil. Other garnishes can include chopped green onions, soy cheese, and salsa.

Vegetables

Kale with Lemon   Serves 4

Kale is one of my favorite vegetables and it also has terrific health benefits for women since it is a good source of calcium and other essential nutrients like lutein which supports the health of your eyes.

1 bunch of kale
1 lemon, cut into quarters
Soy sauce

Rinse kale well and remove stems. Steam for 5-6 minutes or until leaves wilt and are tender. Dress lightly with soy sauce and lemon juice.

Cranberry Almond Brussels Sprouts   Serves 2-4

The dried cranberries in this dish really make it special by adding a touch of tangy sweetness.

2 cups Brussels sprouts, chopped into bite size pieces
2 tablespoons slivered almonds
2 tablespoons dried cranberries, coarsely chopped
1 teaspoon almond oil
Pinch of salt

Steam Brussels sprouts for 5-7 minutes, until slightly tender but retaining their color.

In a frying pan, heat the oil on medium-low. Add almonds and stir until they begin to turn light brown. Add cranberries and continue cooking for 15-30 seconds. Take the pan off the heat and add Brussels sprouts. Cook for a minute and serve.

Jessica's Favorite Broccoli   **Serves 4**

1 pound broccoli
1 tablespoons flax oil
Pinch of salt (optional)
Squeeze of lemon

Cut the broccoli into small flowerets; steam until tender. Squeeze lemon juice over broccoli and add the flax oil. Mix and serve.

Cauliflower with Flax Oil   **Serves 4**

1 medium head cauliflower
2 tablespoons flax oil
Pinch of salt (optional)

Break the cauliflower into small flowerets. Steam until tender. Toss with flax oil and salt.

Roasted Rosemary Potatoes   **Serves 4-6**

I love roasted potatoes! This is a wonderful potato recipe that I like to make when I serve roasted chicken.

4 cups red potatoes – about 4 or 5 large red potatoes
1 tablespoon dried rosemary, crushed
3 tablespoons of olive oil
2 garlic cloves, minced
¼ teaspoon pepper (optional)
Pinch of salt

Preheat oven to 400 degrees. Cut potatoes into bite size pieces and put into plastic bag. Add olive oil, rosemary, garlic, and black pepper to bag. Close bag and shake to coat all of the potato pieces.

Line a baking tray with foil and put potatoes on to tray. Arrange evenly in one layer. Sprinkle salt onto potatoes and bake for 30-35 minutes until brown and cooked through. During cooking stir the potatoes once if desired.

Honey Carrots **Serves 4**

This is one of my favorite side dishes. The warm honey brings out the natural sweetness of the carrots.

3 cups carrots, sliced thin
1 teaspoon honey
1 teaspoon almond oil
Pinch of salt (optional)

Cut carrots into thin slices and steam for 6-8 minutes, or until tender. Using the same saucepan pour out the cooking water and on low heat add the honey and oil and mix well. Add carrots and mix all ingredients together. Add a pinch of salt before serving.

Main Dishes

Mega Greens Rice Bowl   **Serves 4**

This dish is a satisfying way to get a large serving of healthy greens. A delicious sauce is Organicville's Island Teriyaki (organicvillefoods.com). Their sauce is made with agave nectar instead of cane sugar.

4 cups kale, cut into bite size pieces (about ½ bunch)
3 cups baby bok choy, chopped
1 cup of white mushrooms, sliced
1 carrot, finely chopped
8 ounces of tofu, cubed
3 cups cooked brown rice - ¾ cup rice per person
Teriyaki sauce – soy sauce - gomasio

Steam the carrots for 4 minutes and then add the kale, bok choy, mushrooms, and tofu. Steam for 5 minutes. Serve in a deep bowl over rice with your choice of sauce.

Good sauces for this dish include teriyaki sauce and soy sauce. A little bit of lemon juice and gomasio also works well.

Baked Tofu Rice Bowl   Serves 4

Baked tofu has a rich, nutty flavor that I love. This recipe is fun but also very tasty and rich in healthy greens. I always make sure that the vegetables are cut into bite size pieces.

3 cups broccoli, chopped
3 cups baby bok choy, chopped
1 carrot, finely chopped
½ cup mushrooms, sliced
½ cup red pepper
Baked tofu
3 cups cooked brown rice - ¾ cup rice per person

Steam the carrots for 4 minutes and then add the broccoli, baby bok choy, mushrooms, and red pepper. Steam for 5 minutes. Serve in a deep bowl over rice with your choice of sauce. Layer a few pieces of baked tofu on top.

Summertime Veggie Pasta   Serves 4

This light pasta is one of my favorite dishes to eat during the summer. The pasta and sauce are light but filling. It's a dish that I love to share to share with friends.

1 box quinoa elbow pasta (8 ounce box)
½ onion, diced
2 cans Italian seasoned diced tomatoes
1 can garbanzo beans
1 carrot, shredded
1½ cups cooked Brussels sprouts or broccoli
½ teaspoon dried basil
2 teaspoons olive oil
Pinch of pepper
Pinch of salt (optional)

Cook pasta according to package directions. In a saucepan on medium heat add olive oil and onions. Sautee until onions are translucent. Add remainder of ingredients and bring to a simmer. Cook on low heat for 10 minutes. Combine the cooked noodles with the sauce.

Mushroom and Eggplant Sandwich **Serves 2**

This sandwich is a variation on the open-face mushroom sandwich. This sandwich uses eggplant spread instead of mayonnaise and mustard, which gives the sandwich a delightful spiciness. I like the Eggplant Garlic Spread from Trader Joe's. This sandwich is also best served open-face.

4 slices gluten-free bread
4 cups mushrooms, sliced – *I prefer basic white mushrooms*
1½ cups mixed greens
½ tomato, sliced thin
1 teaspoon balsamic vinegar
1 tablespoon olive oil
2 tablespoons eggplant spread
Pinch of salt
Pinch of pepper

Warm a frying pan on medium heat and add olive oil. Add mushrooms and sauté gently adding a generous pinch of salt and pepper. When mushrooms begin to cook down turn heat to low and add balsamic vinegar. Continue to cook until mushrooms are soft and begin to lightly brown. Total cooking time is about 6-8 minutes.

Toast bread and spread on the eggplant spread. Dress each piece of bread with the greens and a slice or two of tomato. Spoon the cooked mushrooms on to each slice of bread.

Parmesan Chicken Pasta **Serves 4**

This dish is a crowd pleaser that I often serve when I have friends over. The Parmesan cheese adds a delightful tanginess that rounds out the dish perfectly.

6 cups gluten-free pasta, cooked
1 ½ cups roasted chicken, cubed
⅔ cup diced carrots
⅔ cup diced red onion
½ onion, diced
1 small tomato, finely chopped
3 cups broccoli, chopped into bite size pieces
⅔ cup chicken broth (recommended) or water
1 teaspoon dried basil
1 tablespoon olive oil
Soy Parmesan cheese or regular, grated
Generous pinch of pepper
Salt (optional)

In a frying pan on medium heat add the olive oil. Add the onion and sauté until the onion begin to turn translucent. Add all vegetables except tomatoes and cook for 1-2 minutes. Add chicken broth, chicken, tomatoes, basil, and pepper. Turn heat to low, cover and simmer for 5-7 minutes or until broth has cooked down. Add more broth if needed.

Add the sauce to the pasta. Serve with Parmesan cheese.

Turkey Bolognese   **Serves 2-4**

This dish cooks up quickly and is very satisfying. This is a versatile recipe. You can add all kinds of vegetables and it will taste great.

½ lb. ground turkey
2 cans of diced tomatoes
1 can tomato paste
½ onion, diced
1 carrot, diced
1 zucchini, diced
1 teaspoon basil
1 teaspoon oregano
1 tablespoon olive oil
¼ teaspoon salt (optional)
½ teaspoon pepper (optional)
Water (optional)

Heat pan on medium and add olive oil. Add onion and sauté until translucent. Add turkey and all herbs and spices. Cook until turkey has browned and cooked thoroughly. Add tomatoes, tomato paste, carrots, and zucchini. Cook on low heat for 12-15 minutes. If sauce is too thick add a small amount of water until desired consistency is reached. Serve over brown rice spaghetti.

Simple Broiled Tuna   **Serves 4**

4 fillets of tuna, 4 ounces each
2 teaspoons olive oil
Squeeze of lemon juice
Pinch of salt

Baste the tuna fillets with oil; then sprinkle with lemon juice. Place tuna in a broiler pan and broil until the level of doneness that you prefer (rare or well-done).

Simple Steamed Salmon   **Serves 4**

4 fillets of salmon, 4 ounces each
1 cup water
Squeeze of lemon

Combine water and lemon juice in a steamer. Place salmon fillets in streamer basket. Cook to the level of doneness that you prefer.

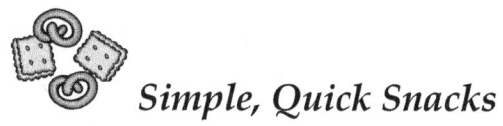 *Simple, Quick Snacks*

Trail Mix   Makes ¾ cup

¼ cup raw unsalted pumpkin seeds
¼ cup raw unsalted sunflower seeds
¼ cup raisins

Combine and store in a container in the refrigerator. This trail mix is very high in essential fatty acids, calcium, magnesium, and iron. I use it for a snack food to replace stressful and unhealthy sugar-based sweets and chocolate. It is a great mix to take on trips, and I eat it often for breakfast.

Rice Cakes with Nut Butter and Jam   Serves 2

4 unsalted rice cakes
2 tablespoons raw almond butter
2 tablespoons fruit preserves (no sugar added)

Spread rice cakes with almond butter and fruit preserves for a quick snack.

Herbal tea makes a good accompaniment.

Rice Cakes with Tuna Fish   Serves 2

4 unsalted rice cakes
4 ounces tuna fish
2 teaspoons low-calorie mayonnaise

Spread rice cakes with tuna fish and mayonnaise. *This is an excellent high-protein, high-carbohydrate snack.*

Apple with Almond Butter   Serves 2

1 apple, sliced
1 tablespoon raw almond butter

Spread almond butter on thin apple slices.

Banana with Sesame Butter   Serves 2

1 banana, halved
1 tablespoon raw sesame butter

Spread sesame butter on each half of a ripe banana.

6

Vitamins, Minerals & Herbs for Menstrual Cramps

Optimal nutrition plays a crucial role in both the treatment and prevention of menstrual pain and cramps. When adequate nutritional support is lacking, I have found it very difficult to entirely relieve cramp symptoms, even with the use of medications. The use of nutritional supplements can help to relieve cramps in many ways. When used properly, they can promote normal muscle tone and relaxation in the pelvic and low back area and relieve pain. They also help to bring blood circulation and oxygen to the pelvic region.

Certain essential nutrients provide the "raw materials" for normal hormone production and balance. In fact, poor or inadequate nutrition may play a major role in causing cramp symptoms. Thus, the use of essential nutrients is an important facet of a good menstrual cramps treatment program. Many research studies done at university centers and hospitals support the importance of nutrition in regulating cramps. I have included a bibliography at the end of this chapter for those wanting more technical information.

The importance of a good diet along with the use of supplements cannot be emphasized too strongly. Supplements are not meant to be used as a rationale to continue poor nutritional habits. I have found that my patients heal most effectively when they combine a nutrient-rich diet with the right mix of supplements. Although nothing can replace a healthful diet, most women have difficulty getting their nutrient intake up to the levels needed for optimal healing through diet alone. The use of supplements can help make up this deficiency so you can heal as rapidly and completely as possible.

This chapter is divided into four sections. The role of vitamins and minerals is discussed in the first section, followed by the beneficial effects of herbs in section two. Section three covers the use of essential fatty acids for menstrual cramps. I complete the chapter with specific recommendations on how to best use nutritional supplements. I have also included a number of helpful food charts that give major food sources for each essential nutrient.

Vitamins and Minerals for Menstrual Cramps

This section describes the numerous vitamins and minerals that can be useful in the treatment and prevention of menstrual cramps. Where possible, I have included optimal doses for the nutrients described. You may find, however, that lower doses work better for you. Start slowly when using supplements and increase your dose gradually until you find the level that works best for you.

Vitamin B-Complex. The B-complex of vitamins consists of eleven factors that work to perform a number of important biochemical functions in the body. These include stabilization of brain chemistry, glucose metabolism, and the inactivation of estrogen by the liver. In fact, vitamin B factors are essential for healthy liver functioning. Emotional and nutritional stress cause loss of the water-soluble B vitamins from the body. Loss of B vitamins can worsen certain symptoms seen with menstrual cramps, including fatigue, faintness, and dizziness. I generally recommend 50 to 100 mg per day of B-complex vitamins. Common food sources of the B-complex vitamins are whole grains, beans and peas, and liver.

Two B vitamins—B3 and B6—are particularly useful for menstrual cramps. Niacin, or vitamin B3, has been shown in clinical research to be effective in relieving 90 percent of menstrual cramps in symptomatic women. The effectiveness of niacin was enhanced with the addition of vitamin C and rutin, a bio-flavonoid. Supplementation needs to be started seven to ten days prior to menses to be effective, and its benefits often remain for several months after stopping its use. Women with pre-existing liver disease should use niacin very cautiously. An optimal dose range for menstrual cramps is 25 to 200 mg per day.

Vitamin B6, or pyridoxine, can be used to help regulate symptoms of both congestive and spasmodic dysmenorrhea. Clinical studies have shown a reduction in cramping, fluid retention, weight gain, and fatigue with the use of B6. An interesting clinical study tested the usefulness of vitamin B6 in decreasing cramps. Women were given vitamin B6 daily throughout the menstrual period as well as during the rest of the month. Duration and intensity of their cramps decreased progressively over a four-to six-month period.

Vitamin B6 is also an important factor in the conversion of linoleic acid to gamma-linolenic acid (GLA) in the production of the beneficial series-1 prostaglandins. Prostaglandins have a relaxant effect on uterine muscles, so they can help to reduce cramps. Vitamin B6 levels are decreased in women using the birth control pill, a common treatment for both spasmodic dysmenorrhea and endometriosis, and should be supplemented. B6 can be safely used in doses up to 300 mg. Doses above this level can be neurotoxic and should be avoided.

Vitamin C. Vitamin C helps increase capillary permeability. This is important for menstrual cramps since it permits better flow of nutrients into the tight and contracted uterine muscle and facilitates the flow of waste products out of the uterus. Waste products that worsen cramping and pain, such as lactic acid and carbon dioxide, are more efficiently released from the pelvic region. Vitamin C is also an important anti-stress vitamin and can help decrease the fatigue and lethargy symptoms that accompany cramps. I recommend that women with cramps use from 500 to 3000 mg of vitamin C per day, especially when symptoms occur.

Vitamin E. Vitamin E has been tested in clinical studies as a treatment for spasmodic dysmenorrhea. It has been used in doses of 150 I.U. ten days premenstrual and during the first four days of the menstrual period. It helped to relieve symptoms of menstrual discomfort within two menstrual cycles in approximately 70 percent of the women tested. Vitamin E has a powerful effect on the hormonal system. It has also been used to reduce breast tenderness, fibrocystic disease of the breast, and PMS symptoms, as well as hot flashes in menopausal women. It is obviously a very important nutrient for women's health. The best natural sources of vitamin E are wheat germ oil, walnut oil, soy bean oil, and other grain and seed oil sources. I generally recommend that women with cramps use from 400 to 800 I.U. per day. Women with hypertension and diabetes should start on a much lower dose of vitamin E (100 I.U./day). Any increase in dosage should be made slowly and monitored carefully in these women. Otherwise, vitamin E tends to be extremely safe and is commonly used by millions of men and women.

Calcium. This important mineral helps to prevent menstrual cramps by maintaining normal muscle tone. When taken before bed at night, it is also effective in helping to combat insomnia due to menstrual discomfort. Muscles that are calcium-deficient tend to be hyperactive and more likely to cramp. Since the uterus is made up of muscle, it is susceptible to calcium deficiency. Besides its role in promoting normal muscle tone and activity, calcium is also a major structural component of the bones. Unfortunately, calcium deficiency is common in our society. The recommended daily allowance (RDA) for calcium in menstruating women is 800 mg per day and rises to as much as 1500 mg per day in postmenopausal women. The typical American diet supplies only about 450 to 550 mg per day. No wonder so many American women are at risk for menstrual cramps and osteoporosis. Good food sources of calcium include green leafy vegetables, beans and peas, seeds and nuts, blackstrap molasses, and seafood.

Magnesium. Magnesium has an important effect on the neuromuscular system in reducing menstrual cramps. Like calcium, a deficiency of magnesium increases muscular hyperactivity. Magnesium optimizes the amount of usable calcium in your system by increasing calcium absorption. Conversely, calcium can interfere with magnesium absorption. Magnesium deficiency also worsens menstrual fatigue, dizziness, and fainting because of its importance in glucose metabolism.

A magnesium deficiency can hinder the normal conversion of food to usable energy. Magnesium is also needed for the conversion of linoleic acid to gamma-linolenic acid (GLA). Like vitamin B6, a deficiency of magnesium retards the conversion of essential fatty acids to the series-1 prostaglandins. Like calcium, magnesium is also an important structural component of healthy bone tissue. It is necessary for the prevention of osteoporosis. It is usually recommended that the diet include half as much magnesium as calcium, or approximately 400 mg per day. Most women get only one-third to one-half of that amount in their daily diet. This puts them at high risk of menstrual cramping and pain.

Iron. Women who have iron deficiency anemia may be at higher risk of menstrual cramps because of the diminished oxygen-carrying capability of the red blood cells. One interesting clinical study showed that when the iron deficiency anemia was resolved, the menstrual cramping disappeared. Young women in their teens and twenties are not only very prone to iron deficiency, but they are also at the peak age for spasmodic dysmenorrhea. Teenagers are prone to heavier menstrual flows during the first few years after they begin menstruation. Also, teenagers and young women in their twenties often eat an iron-poor diet, full of fat and sugar. The RDA for iron is 15 mg. Good food sources of iron include blackstrap molasses, seafood, eggs, liver, vegetables, seeds, nuts, beans, and peas.

Herbs for Menstrual Cramps

A wide variety of herbs will alleviate menstrual cramp symptoms. I have used various cramp-relieving herbs in my practice and many of my patients have found them to be gentle, effective remedies. I use them as a form of extended nutrition, a way of balancing and expanding the diet and optimizing nutritional intake. Some herbs provide an additional source of essential nutrients such as calcium, magnesium, and potassium that help to relieve cramps. Other herbs actually have mild relaxant, diuretic, and anti-inflammatory properties aside from their nutritional content; these help to relieve painful symptoms with a minimum of side effects.

In Traditional Chinese Medicine, cramps are considered a yang condition worsened by an excess of foods such as meat and salt. These foods are thought to have a contracting effect on the body. In this practice, cramps are treated by special herbs that have a contrary yin effect and cause muscle relaxation and blood vessel dilation. In this section, I describe many specific herbs useful for the reduction of menstrual cramp symptoms.

Sedative Herbs. Herbs such as valerian root, passion flower, hops, and chamomile have a significant calming and restful effect on the central nervous system. They all promote muscle relaxation as well as emotional calm and well-being. With their mild sedative effect, they also promote restful sleep, a state that is difficult to induce when a woman is suffering from menstrual pain.

Passion flower has been found to elevate levels of the neurotransmitter serotonin. Serotonin is synthesized from tryptophan, an essential amino acid that has been shown in numerous medical studies to initiate restful sleep. Chamomile, an herb that makes delicate, tasty tea, is a good source of tryptophan. Valerian root has been used extensively in traditional herbal medicine as a sleep inducer and is widely used both in Europe and the United States as a gentle herbal remedy to help combat insomnia. Unfortunately, valerian has an unpleasant taste, making it more palatable when used in capsule form. Both valerian root and chamomile are also effective in relieving indigestion and intestinal gas. Hops and peppermint are other soothing herbs that can be used as teas.

Muscle-Relaxant Herbs. Several Chinese herbs have been used for thousands of years for the treatment of menstrual cramps because they have a direct relaxant effect on the uterine muscle. These herbs are generally available in the United States in health food stores and Chinese herbal shops. Dong quai, or angelica sinensis, is considered an important and effective relaxant herb in Traditional Chinese Medicine. Angelica root extracts cause an initial increase in uterine tension and contraction, which is then followed by relaxation. Angelica also has significant pain-relieving properties as well, rivaling the effectiveness of aspirin.

Peony root is often used in combination with angelica in the treatment of menstrual cramps; it has similar physiological effects on the uterine muscle, but its relaxant effect is more pronounced. Cramp bark is an American herb often used to treat menstrual cramps. It contains vitamin C and may help to relax the muscle by improving capillary permeability, which aids the flow of essential nutrients to the tense muscle and helps remove the waste products that can worsen cramping, such as lactic acid. Black cohosh has a long history in American herbology as effective remedy for menstrual cramps. Recent studies have confirmed its efficacy in relieving menstrual pain. I have used these herbs often with patients who have noted significant relief of menstrual discomfort.

Anti-Inflammatory Herbs. White willow contains an active painkilling chemical bark called salicin which was isolated around 1828 by French and German chemists. Years later, salicylic acid, the pre-cursor of aspirin, was purified. Another natural source of this aspirin precursor was discovered in the herb meadowsweet. Both meadow-sweet and white willow bark reduce inflammation, pain, and fever. They can be used effectively to help treat menstrual cramps and menstrual headaches since they are able to suppress the action of the series-2 prostaglandins. Unfortunately, like aspirin, they can produce the unwanted side effects of gastric indigestion, nausea, and diarrhea, so use these herbs carefully. In contrast, both ginger and bromelain, a natural digestive aid found in pineapple, effectively suppress series-2 prostaglandins without the harmful side effects.

Diuretic Herbs. Many herbs act as mild diuretic agents. They can be useful in the treatment of primary congestive dysmenorrhea by reducing bloating and fluid retention. I have used many of them in my practice as mild teas or in tincture form. Some of the most commonly used herbs for congestive symptoms include buchu, celery, dandelion, horsetail, parsley, nettle, sarsaparilla, and uva ursi. All the herbs with diuretic action can deplete your potassium stores on a long-term basis, though they are still much milder than the prescription diuretics. If you use these herbs on a regular basis to treat or prevent primary congestive dysmenorrhea, be sure to eat foods that are high in potassium such as bananas, oranges, raw seeds, and most fruits, as well as nuts and fresh vegetables.

Blood-Circulation Enhancers. Herbs such as ginger and ginkgo biloba improve circulation to the pelvis and lower extremities. Ginger causes a widening of the blood vessels. Better blood circulation helps to draw nutrients to the contracted uterus and low back muscles and also helps to remove waste products like lactic acid and carbon dioxide. Ginger also has an antispasmodic effect on the smooth muscle of the intestinal tract and can help to relieve the digestive symptoms that occur with menstrual cramps, including nausea, vomiting, and bowel changes. (Its benefits as a series-2 prostaglandin inhibitor are mentioned above.) Ginger is obviously a useful herb for women with menstrual cramps.

Besides taking ginger in tincture or capsule form, you can also use it as a delicious tea. To make ginger tea, buy a fresh ginger root from your local supermarket. Grate a few teaspoons of the fresh root into a quart pot of water. Boil and steep for 30 minutes. This is a very soothing herbal tea, delicious with a small amount of honey.

Ginkgo biloba improves blood circulation and oxygenation to the pelvic region and lower extremities. It has a vasodilating effect and also decreases metabolic processes during a period of decreased blood supply. It is a very powerful herbal remedy and can be effectively combined with ginger.

Essential Fatty Acids for Menstrual Cramps

Sufficient essential fatty acids are an extremely important part of the nutritional program for any women with menstrual cramps, whether caused by spasmodic dysmenorrhea or endometriosis. As mentioned earlier in the book, essential fatty acids are the raw materials from which the beneficial hormone-like chemicals called prostaglandins are made. The prostaglandins from essential fatty acids help to reduce uterine spasms and relax blood vessels. This can significantly reduce muscle cramps and tension.

There are two essential fatty acids, linoleic acid (omega-6 family) and alpha-linolenic acid (omega-3 family). They are derived from specific food sources in our diet, primarily raw seeds and nuts. EPA (eicosapentaenoic acid) and DHA (docosahexaenoic acid) are members of the omega-3 family and are found in certain fish including salmon, mackerel, and trout. Linoleic and alpha-linolenic acids cannot be made by the body and must be supplied daily in our diets, from either food or supplements. However, once these fatty acids are supplied in the diet, some women may lack the ability to convert them efficiently to the series-1 and series-3 prostaglandins which help to prevent menstrual cramps and bloating. For example, linoleic acid, which must be converted to a chemical called gamma-linolenic acid (GLA) on its way to becoming the series-1 prostaglandin.

The conversion of linoleic acid to GLA requires the presence of magnesium, vitamin B6, zinc, vitamin C, and niacin. Women who are deficient in these nutrients can't make the chemical conversions effectively. In addition, women who eat a high-cholesterol diet, eat processed oils such as mayonnaise, use a great deal of alcohol, or are diabetic may find the fatty acid conversion to the series-1 prostaglandin difficult to achieve. Other factors that impede prostaglandin production include emotional stress, allergies, and eczema. In women with these risk factors, less than 1 percent of linoleic acid may be converted to GLA. The rest of the fatty acids can be used as an energy source, but they will not be able to play a role in relieving menstrual cramp symptoms.

Studies have been done on essential fatty acids as a treatment for PMS. Women with PMS often have the congestive type of dysmenorrhea with bloating, weight gain, and dull aching pain in the pelvic region. These studies have shown that the use of essential fatty acids can reduce most PMS symptoms by as much as 70 percent. Evening primrose oil, borage oil, and black currant oil are the most common supplemental sources of essential fatty acid for the treatment of cramps and PMS. All three oils contain high levels of GLA, allowing women to circumvent the difficult conversion process of linoleic acid to GLA. In addition, a recent study also found that fish oil, a precursor of the series-3 prostaglandins, was very useful in reducing menstrual cramps.

The best food sources of essential fatty acids are flaxseeds and chia seeds which contain high levels of both linoleic and linolenic acid. Both the seeds and their oils can be used and should be absolutely fresh and unspoiled. Because these oils become rancid when exposed to light and air (oxygen), they need to be packed in special opaque containers and kept in the refrigerator. Fresh flaxseed oil is my special favorite. It is available in health food stores. Flax oil is golden, rich, and delicious. It is extremely high in linoleic and alpha-linolenic acids, which comprise about 70 percent of its total content. Flax oil has a wonderful flavor and can be used as a butter replacement on foods such as mashed potatoes, popcorn, steamed broccoli, cauliflower, carrots, and bread. Flax oil (and all other essential oils) should never be used in cooking, as heat affects the special chemical properties of these oils. Instead, add these oils as a form of flavoring to foods that are already cooked.

Chia seeds are also a great and very well balanced source of both alpha-linolenic acid and linoleic acid. In addition, they are an excellent source of vegetable protein, giber, complex carbohydrates and antioxidants. Not only are they beneficial in relieving menstrual cramps and pain but they help to stabilize your blood sugar level, reduce your craving for sugary and refined carbohydrate foods and improves your mental focus. These additional benefits are also very helpful in promoting great health in midlife and beyond. You can eat up to 1 ounce of chia seeds each day.

Omega-3 fatty acids are also found in abundance in fish oils. The best sources are cold-water, high-fat fish such as salmon, tuna, rainbow trout, mackerel, and eel. These oils are excellent for preventing and healing menstrual cramps and pain. Omega-3 rich fish can be eaten once or twice a week at most because of the high levels of mercury currently contaminating fish. I recommend for daily use that you use fish oil capsules containing 1500 to 2000 mg of the omega-3 fatty acids total per day.

Linoleic acid (omega-6 family) by itself can be found in seeds and seed oils. Good sources include safflower oil, sunflower oil, corn oil, sesame seed oil, and wheat germ oil. Many women prefer to use fresh raw sesame seeds, sunflower seeds, and wheat germ to obtain the oils. The average healthy adult requires only four teaspoons per day of the essential oils in their diet, although women with menstrual cramps may need several tablespoons per day of the fresh oil. If you use the whole flaxseed, remember that the seeds are 50 percent oil by content, so you need twice as much whole seed intake as oil to obtain the same amount of fatty acids. For optimal results, be sure to use these oils along with vitamin E. The vitamin E also helps to prevent rancidity of the oils.

Nutritional Supplements for Women with Menstrual Cramps

Good dietary habits are crucial for control of your menstrual cramp symptoms. But for many women, the use of nutritional supplements is important in order to achieve high levels of the essential nutrients needed to heal menstrual cramps. On the following pages is a sample of the vitamins and minerals as well as their dosages that can be used as a foundation for your program. You can also add the other nutrients like flaxseed oil and fish oil that I have discussed in this chapter to fill out your program. You may find it easier to implement your program if you start with one of the better quality multi-nutrient products for women that are available in health food stores and through the internet and then add the remaining essential nutrients.

Remember that all women differ somewhat in their nutritional needs. If you do take the recommended vitamin or herbal supplements, I usually advise that you start with one-fourth to one-half the dose recommended in this book and work your way up slowly to the higher dosage, if needed. You may find that you do best with slightly more or less of certain ingredients. I recommend that patients take their supplements with meals or at least a snack. Very rarely, a woman will have a digestive reaction to supplements, such as nausea or indigestion. If this happens, stop all supplements; then resume using them, adding one at a time, until you find the offending nutrient. Eliminate from your program any nutrient to which you have a reaction. If you have any specific questions, ask a health-care professional who is knowledgeable about nutrition.

Optional Nutritional Supplementation for Menstrual Cramps

Vitamins and Minerals

Vitamin A	5000 I.U.
Beta-carotene (provitamin A)	5,000 – 25,000 I.U.
Vitamin B-complex	
B1 (thiamine)	25 - 100 mg
B2 (riboflavin)	25 - 100 mg
B3 (niacinamide)	25 - 100 mg
B5 (pantothenic acid)	25 - 100 mg
B6 (pyridoxine)	50 – 100 mg
B12 (cyanocobalamin)	100 – 750 mcg
Folic acid	400 – 800 mcg
Biotin	200 - 500 mcg
Choline	25 - 100 mg
Inositol	25 - 100 mg
PABA	25 - 100 mg
Vitamin C (as mineral ascorbates)	1000-2000 mg
Vitamin D	1000 I.U.
Bioflavonoids	800-2000 mg
Rutin	200 mg
Vitamin E (d-alpha tocopherol acetate)	800-1600 I.U.
Calcium	1000 - 1200 mg
Magnesium	500 - 600 mg
Potassium	100 mg
Iron	18 mg
Zinc	15 mg
Iodine	150 mcg
Manganese	5 mg
Copper	2 mg
Selenium	200 mcg
Chromium	100 – 200 mcg
Boron	3 mg

Summary Chart For Nutritional Supplements

I want to end this section by summarizing the nutritional supplements that you can take to help eliminate your menstrual cramps. These include:

1. **Vitamins and Minerals** - Vitamin B-Complex, Vitamin C, Vitamin E, Calcium, Magnesium, and Iron.

2. **Herbs** – valerian root, passion flower, hops, chamomile, dong quai, angelica root, peony root, cramp bark, black cohosh, meadow-sweet bark, white willow bark, buchu, celery, dandelion, horsetail, parsley, nettle, sarsaparilla, uva ursi, ginger and ginkgo biloba.

3. **Essential Fatty Acids** - Linoleic acid (omega-6 family) and alpha-linolenic acid (omega-3 family). The best sources of omega-6 fatty acids are evening primrose oil, borage oil, and black currant oil. The best source of omega-3 fatty acids are flaxseeds, chia seeds and fish oil (EPA and DHA) from cold water, high-fat fish such as salmon, tuna, rainbow trout, mackerel, and eel.

Food Sources of Vitamin A

Vegetables	*Fruits*	*Meat, poultry, seafood*
Carrots	Apricots	Crab
Carrot juice	Avocado	Halibut
Collard greens	Cantaloupe	Liver — all types
Dandelion greens	Mangoes	Mackerel
Green onions	Papaya	Salmon
Kale	Peaches	Swordfish
Parsley	Persimmons	
Spinach		
Sweet potatoes		
Turnip greens		
Winter squash		

Food Sources of Vitamin B-Complex (including folic acid)

Vegetables	*Legumes*	*Grains*
Alfalfa	Garbanzo beans	Barley
Artichoke	Lentils	Bran
Asparagus	Lima beans	Brown rice
Beets	Pinto beans	Corn Millet
Broccoli	Soybeans	Rice bran
Brussels sprouts		Wheat
Cabbage	*Meat, poultry, seafood*	Wheat germ
Cauliflower	Egg yolks*	
Green beans	Liver*	*Sweeteners*
Kale		Blackstrap molasses
Leeks	*Eggs and meat should be*	
Onions	*from organic, range-free*	
Peas	*stock fed on pesticide-free*	
Romaine lettuce	*food.*	

Food Sources of Vitamin B6

Grains	Vegetables	Meat, poultry, seafood
Brown rice	Asparagus	Chicken
Buckwheat flour	Beet greens	Salmon
Rice bran	Broccoli	Shrimp
Rye flour	Brussels sprouts	Tuna
Wheat germ	Cauliflower	
Whole wheat flour	Green peas	*Nuts and seeds*
	Leeks	Sunflower seeds
	Sweet potatoes	

Food Sources of Vitamin C

Fruits	Vegetables and legumes	Meat, poultry, seafood
Blackberries	Asparagus	Liver—all types
Black currants	Black-eyed peas	Pheasant
Cantaloupe	Broccoli	Quail
Elderberries	Brussels sprouts	Salmon
Grapefruit	Cabbage	
Grapefruit juice	Cauliflower	
Guavas	Collards	
Kiwi fruit	Green onions	
Mangoes	Green peas	
Oranges	Kale	
Orange juice	Kohlrabi	
Pineapple	Parsley	
Raspberries	Potatoes	
Strawberries	Rutabagas	
Tangerines	Sweet pepper	
Tomatoes	Sweet potatoes	
	Turnips	

Food Sources of Vitamin E

Vegetables
Asparagus
Cucumber
Green peas
Kale

Nuts and seeds
Almonds
Brazil nuts
Hazelnuts
Peanuts

Meats, poultry, seafood
Haddock
Herring
Mackerel
Lamb
Liver — all types

Oils
Corn
Peanut
Safflower
Sesame
Soybean
Wheat germ

Grains
Brown rice
Millet

Fruits
Mangoes

Food Sources of Essential Fatty Acids

Oils
Flax
Pumpkin
Soybean

Walnut
Safflower
Sunflower

Grape
Corn
Wheat germ
Sesame

Food Sources of Iron

Grains
Bran cereal (All-Bran)
Bran muffin
Millet, dry
Oat flakes
Pasta, whole wheat
Pumpernickel bread
Wheat germ

Legumes
Black beans
Black-eyed peas
Garbanzo beans
Kidney beans
Lentils
Lima beans
Pinto beans
Soybeans
Split peas
Tofu

Vegetables
Beets
Beet greens
Broccoli
Brussels sprouts
Corn
Dandelion greens
Green beans
Kale
Leeks
Spinach
Sweet potatoes
Swiss chard

Fruits
Apple juice
Avocado
Blackberries
Dates, dried
Figs
Prunes, dried
Prune juice
Raisins

Meat, poultry, seafood
Beef liver
Calf's liver
Chicken liver
Clams
Oysters
Sardines
Scallops
Trout

Nuts and seeds
Almonds
Pecans
Pistachios
Sesame butter
Sesame seeds
Sunflower seeds

Food Sources of Calcium

Vegetables and legumes
Artichoke
Black beans
Black-eyed peas
Beet greens
Broccoli
Brussels sprouts
Cabbage
Collards
Eggplant
Garbanzo beans
Green beans
Green onions
Kale
Kidney beans
Leeks
Lentils
Parsley
Parsnips
Pinto beans
Rutabagas
Soybeans
Spinach
Turnips
Watercress

Meat, poultry, seafood
Abalone
Beef
Bluefish
Carp
Crab
Haddock
Herring
Lamb
Lobster
Oysters
Perch
Salmon
Shrimp
Venison

Fruits
Blackberries
Black currants
Boysenberries
Oranges
Pineapple juice
Prunes
Raisins
Rhubarb
Tangerine juice

Grains
Bran
Brown rice
Bulgar wheat
Millet

Food Sources of Magnesium

Vegetables and legumes
Artichoke
Black-eyed peas
Carrot juice
Corn
Green peas
Leeks
Lima beans
Okra
Parsnips
Potatoes
Soybean sprouts
Spinach
Squash
Yams
Snapper
Turkey
Papaya

Meat, poultry, seafood
Beef
Carp
Chicken
Clams
Cod
Crab
Duck
Haddock
Herring
Lamb
Mackerel
Oysters
Salmon
Shrimp
Raisins
Prunes

Nuts and seeds
Almonds
Brazil nuts
Hazelnuts
Peanuts
Pistachios
Pumpkin seeds
Sesame seeds
Walnuts

Fruits
Avocado
Banana
Grapefruit juice
Pineapple juice

Grains
Millet
Brown rice
Wild rice

Food Sources of Potassium

Vegetables and legumes	Meat, poultry, seafood	Nuts and seeds
Artichoke	Bass	Almonds
Asparagus	Beef	Brazil nuts
Black-eyed peas	Carp	Chestnuts
Beets	Catfish	Hazelnuts
Brussels sprouts	Chicken	Macadamia nuts
Carrot juice	Cod	Peanuts
Cauliflower	Duck	Pistachios
Corn	Eel	Pumpkin seeds
Garbanzo beans	Flatfish	Sesame seeds
Green beans	Haddock	Sunflower seeds
Kidney beans	Halibut	Walnuts
Leeks	Herring	
Lentils	Lamb	*Fruits*
Lima beans	Lobster	Apricots
Navy beans	Mackerel	Avocado
Okra	Oysters	Banana
Parsnips	Perch	Cantaloupe
Peas	Pike	Currants
Pinto beans	Salmon	Figs
Potatoes	Scallops	Grapefruit juice
Pumpkin	Shrimp	Orange juice
Soybean sprouts	Snapper	Papaya
Spinach	Trout	Pineapple juice
Squash	Turkey	Prunes
Yams	Raisins	
		Grains
		Brown rice
		Millet
		Wild rice

7

Stress Reduction for Menstrual Cramps

Emotional stress can be a significant trigger for pain, discomfort, and muscle tension. Though we can't always avoid significant stress in our life, we can modify its physical and psychological effects.

The pace of life in Western societies reinforces the tendency toward muscle tension and cramping in sensitive women. To feel rushed and tense is typical in our goal-oriented culture; everything seems to be done in a hurry and on deadlines. We may feel a continual sense of urgency to meet a particular set of goals without giving much attention to how to reach those goals. As a reaction to this sense of urgency, our bodies may tense unconsciously.

Exercises for stress reduction can be a very important part of your menstrual cramp self-help program. For many women, the intensity of menstrual cramps varies from month to month. My patients frequently tell me that their cramps are worse when they are more upset. As you begin to anticipate the onset of your menstrual period and cramps, I recommend using stress-reduction techniques on a daily basis. They can really make a difference. If you break up the tasks of the day with a few minutes of stress-reducing exercises, you will feel much more relaxed. With the use of these stress-reduction techniques, you can still accomplish the tasks on time but in a much more relaxed, enjoyable, and health-enhancing manner.

Techniques for Relaxation

To help you deal with the emotional stresses that may become magnified in intensity if you are suffering from menstrual cramps and low back pain, I recommend a variety of relaxation methods. These include focusing, meditation, affirmations, and visualizations. All these methods can help to promote a sense of calm and well-being if practiced on a regular basis. In this chapter, I have included exercises from all these categories for you to try. Choose those you enjoy most and practice them on a regular basis. I have taught these exercises to women patients for many years and love to practice them myself. I usually recommend that my patients learn these techniques on their own through books and tapes, but I sometimes go over the exercises with patients at my office. My patients have been very enthusiastic about the results that they attain through stress-reduction exercises. They often feel much calmer and happier, and also find their physical health is improved. A calm mind seems to have beneficial effects on the body's physiology and chemistry, producing a normalizing effect.

To prepare yourself for the relaxation exercises in this chapter, I suggest that you take the following steps:

First Step. Find a comfortable position. For many women, this means lying on their backs. You may also do the exercises sitting up. Try to keep your spine as straight as possible. Your arms and legs should be uncrossed. It is important that your clothes be loose and comfortable.

Second Step. Focus your attention upon the exercises so that distracting thoughts do not interfere with your concentration. Close your eyes and take a few deep breaths, in and out. This will help to remove your thoughts from the problems and tasks of the day and begin to quiet your mind.

The next exercises will help you to get in touch with your own areas of muscle tension and then teach you how to release this tension. This is an important sequence for women with chronic menstrual cramps, low back pain, and abdominal discomfort, because all these symptoms are due in part to chronically tight and tense muscles. Tense muscles tend to have decreased blood circulation and oxygenation and accumulate an excess of waste products such as carbon dioxide and lactic acid.

Interestingly enough, some women with cramps and pelvic pain tend to be habitually tense in these areas throughout the month, even during the time when menstrual cramps are absent. Often they have a tendency to tighten the pelvis and lower abdominal muscles as a stress response to a variety of work, relationship, and sexual stresses. Usually, this muscular tensing of the pelvic muscles is an unconscious response that develops over many years and sets up the emotional patterning that triggers cramps.

For example, when a woman has uptight and uncomfortable feelings about sex or a particular sexual partner, she may tighten these muscles when engaging in or even thinking about sex. Tense muscles also affect a woman's moods, making her more "uptight" and irritable. Muscular and emotional tension usually coexist. Movement is one effective way to break up these habitual patterns of muscle holding and contracting. When muscles are loose and limber, a woman tends to feel more relaxed and in a better mood. Anxiety tends to fade away, being replaced by a sense of expansiveness and calm.

Exercise 1: Focusing

If you have menstrual cramps and low back pain, this focusing exercise allows you to take your attention off the pelvic region and lower part of your body and place your focus elsewhere. By clearing your mind along with doing deep breathing, you may find at the end of this exercise that your discomfort level has diminished in severity.

- Sit upright in a comfortable position.

- Hold several coins, such as 2 quarters, in the palm of your hand.

- Focus all your attention on these coins.

- Inhale and exhale as you do this. Continue to concentrate for 30 seconds. Don't let any other thoughts enter your mind. At the end of this time, notice your breathing. You will probably find that it has slowed down and is calmer. You will probably feel a sense of peacefulness and a decrease in any anxiety that you had before beginning this exercise.

Exercise 2: Discovering Muscle Tension

- Lie on your back in a comfortable position. Allow your arms to rest comfortably at your sides, palms down, on the surface next to you.

- Now, raise just the right hand and arm and hold it elevated for 15 seconds.

- Notice if your forearm feels tight and tense or if the muscles are soft and pliable.

- Now, let your hand and arm drop down and relax. The arm muscles will relax too.

- As you lie still, notice any other parts of your body that feel tense, muscles that feel tight and sore. You may notice a constant dull aching in certain muscles. Tense muscles block blood flow and cut off the supply of nutrients to the tissues. In response to the poor oxygenation, the muscle produces lactic acid, which further worsens muscular discomfort.

Exercise 3: Progressive Muscle Relaxation

- Lie on your back in a comfortable position. Allow your arms to rest at your sides, palms down, on the surface next to you.

- Inhale and exhale slowly and deeply

- Clench your hands into fists and hold them tightly for 15 seconds. As you do this, relax the rest of your body. Visualize your fists contracting, becoming tighter and tighter.

- Then let your hands relax. On relaxing, see a golden light flowing into the entire body, making all your muscles soft and pliable.

- Now, tense and relax the following parts of your body in this order: face, shoulders, back, stomach, pelvis, legs, feet, and toes. Hold each part tensed for 15 seconds and then relax your body for 30 seconds before going on to the next part.

- Finish the exercise by shaking your hands and imagining the remaining tension flowing out of your fingertips.

Exercise 4: Healing Meditation

This exercise provides a healing meditation through a series of positive images. The mind and body are inextricably linked. When you visualize a beautiful scene in which your body is being healed, you actually stimulate positive chemical and hormonal changes in your body that help to create this condition. Likewise, if you visualize a negative scene, such as a fight with a spouse or boss, the negative mental picture can actually trigger an output of chemicals from your body that can worsen pain and discomfort. The axiom that we are what we think is literally true. I have seen the power of positive thinking for years in my medical practice. I always tell my patients that it is much harder to heal the body if the mind is full of upsetting, angry, or fearful images. I have found that healing meditations, when practiced on a regular basis, can be a powerful tool for healing.

- Lie on your back in a comfortable position. Inhale and exhale slowly and deeply.

- Visualize a beautiful green meadow full of lovely fragrant flowers. In the middle of this meadow is a golden temple. See the temple emanating peace and healing.

- Visualize yourself entering this temple. You are the only person inside. It is still and peaceful. As you stand inside of this temple, you feel a healing energy fill every pore of your body with a warm golden light. This energy feels like a healing balm that relaxes you totally. All anxiety dissolves and fades from your mind. You feel completely at ease.

- Open your eyes and continue breathing deeply and slowly for a few more cycles.

Exercise 5: Peaceful Meditation

Meditation requires you to sit quietly and engage in a simple and repetitive activity. By emptying your mind, you give yourself a rest. The metabolism of your body slows down. The brain wave slows from the fast beta wave that predominates during our normal working day to a slower alpha or theta wave. This slower pattern is what appears during sleep or in the period of deep relaxation just prior to falling asleep. Meditating gives your mind a break from tension and worry. It is useful to do during menstruation when every little stress is magnified. After meditating you may wonder what all your upset was about. You will see that situations are not as bad as you believed them to be.

- Lie or sit in a comfortable position.

- Close your eyes and breathe deeply. Let your breathing be slow and relaxed.

- Focus all your attention on your breathing. Notice the movement of your chest and abdomen in and out.

- Block out all other thoughts, feelings, and sensations. If you feel your attention wandering, bring it back to your breathing.

- Say the word "peace" as you inhale. Say the word "calm" as you exhale. Draw out the pronunciation of the word so that it lasts for the entire breath. The word "peace" sounds like: p-e-e-e-a-a-ac-c-c-e-e-e. The word "calm" sounds like: c-a-a-a-l-l-l-m-m-m. Repeating these two words will help you to concentrate.

- Repeat this exercise until you feel very relaxed.

Exercise 6: Affirmations

Affirmations are very important because they align your mind with your body in a positive way. Just as the preceding healing meditation achieved this goal through the use of positive images, affirmations do it through the power of suggestion. Your state of health is determined in part by the interaction between your mind and body via the thousands of messages you send yourself each day with your thoughts. It is not enough to follow an excellent diet and a vigorous exercise routine when you are in the process of healing menstrual cramps. You must tell your body that it is a well, fully functional system. I have seen people stay ill because they sabotage their healing program by sending themselves a barrage of negative messages.

You can aggravate your menstrual cramps and discomfort with negative thoughts because when your body believes it is sick, it behaves accordingly. Thus, it is essential that you cultivate a positive belief system and a positive body image as part of your healing program.

Sit in a comfortable position. Repeat the following affirmations. Repeat those that are particularly important to you 3 times.

- My female system is strong and healthy

- My hormones are balanced and normal.

- My hormonal levels are perfectly regulated.

- My body chemistry is balanced and normal.

- I go through my monthly menstrual cycle with ease and comfort.

- My body feels wonderful as I start each monthly period.

- I barely know that my body is getting ready to menstruate.

- I feel wonderful each month before I menstruate.

- My uterus is relaxed and receptive; I welcome my monthly period.

- My low back muscles feel supple and pliable with each menstrual cycle.

- I am relaxed and at ease as my period approaches.

- I desire a well-balanced and healthful diet.

- I eat only the foods that are good for my body.

- It is a real pleasure to take good care of my body.

- I love my body; I feel at ease in my body.

- My body is pain-free and relaxed.

- I do the level of exercise that keeps my body healthy and supple.

- I handle stress easily and in a relaxed manner.

Exercise 7: Visualizations

Visualization exercises help you to lay down the mental blueprint for a healthier body. This powerful visual technique can actually stimulate positive chemical and hormonal changes in your body that help create the desired outcome. You are literally imaging your body the way you want it to be. Visualization has been used to great benefit by patients with many types of illnesses. It was pioneered by Carl Simonton, M.D., a cancer radiation therapist, who used this technique with his patients. Instead of seeing their cancers as "big destructive monsters," Dr. Simonton had his patients see their immune systems as big white knights or white sharks attacking the small and insignificant cancer cells and destroying them (instead of the other way around). In a substantial number of cases, he saw his patients' health improve.

Visualization exercises can also help to modify your behavior so that you can create the positive body images that you like. With the practice of visualization, you are more likely to choose your foods carefully and practice regular exercise programs to help your body fit the desired images.

Visualizing the following scene should take a minute or two. Linger on any images that particularly please you.

- Close your eyes. Begin to breathe deeply. Inhale and let the air out slowly. Feel your body begin to relax.

- Imagine that you can look, as if through a magic mirror, deep inside your body.

- Look at your female organs. See your uterus and ovaries. They are an attractive pink color. Your uterus is relaxed and supple. It has good blood circulation. Visualize blood flow and oxygen bringing nourishment to the uterus. See waste products flowing out of the uterus and back into the blood circulation to be removed from the body.

- See your ovaries. They are extremely healthy and produce just the right levels of hormones. They are shiny and pink and look like two almonds. The fallopian tubes that pick up the eggs and bring them to the uterus are open, elastic, and expandable. They are totally open and healthy.

- Look at your abdominal and low back muscles. They are soft and pliable with a healthy muscle tone. They are relaxed and free of tension during your menstrual period. Your abdomen is flat, yet the area feels relaxed. Your fluid balance is perfect in your pelvic area.

- Look at your entire body and enjoy the sense of peace and calm running through your body. You feel wonderful.

- Now stop visualizing the scene and focus on your deep breathing, inhaling and exhaling slowly.

- You open your eyes and feel very good.

More Stress-Reduction Techniques for Menstrual Cramps

The rest of this chapter contains additional techniques that I have found over the years to be very useful for relaxation of tight and tense muscles. These methods are also useful in inducing deep emotional relaxation. Try them for a delightful experience.

Hydrotherapy

For centuries, people have used warm water as a way to relax muscles and calm moods. You can have your own "spa" at home by adding relaxing ingredients to the bathwater. I have found the following recipes to be extremely useful in relieving muscle pain and tension.

Recipe 1: Alkaline Bath. Run a tub of warm water. Heat will increase your menstrual flow, so keep the water a little cooler if heavy flow is a problem. Add one cup of sea salt and one cup of bicarbonate of soda to the tub. This is a highly alkaline mixture and I recommend using it only once or twice a month. I've found it very helpful in reducing cramps and calming anxiety and irritability. Soak for 20 minutes. You will probably feel very relaxed and sleepy after this bath; use it at night before going to sleep. You will probably wake up feeling refreshed and energized the following day. Heat of any kind helps to release muscle tension. You may also want to try a hot water bottle or a heating pad to relieve cramps.

Recipe 2: Hydrogen Peroxide Bath. This is one of my personal favorites. Hydrogen peroxide is a combination of water and oxygen, so by adding it to your bath, you are using it to "hyper-oxygenate" your bathwater. Hydrogen peroxide is inexpensive and can be purchased from your local drug store. I usually add three pint bottles of the 3-percent solution to a full tub of warm water and soak for up to a half-hour. If you use the stronger food or technical-grade hydrogen peroxide (35-percent strength), you need to add only 6 ounces. With the more concentrated peroxide, be sure to avoid direct contact with your hands or eyes, and keep it stored in a cool place as it is a very powerful oxidizer.

Sound

Music can have a tremendously relaxing effect on our minds and bodies. For women with menstrual cramps and low back pain, I recommend slow, quiet music—classical music is particularly good. This type of music can have a pronounced beneficial effect on your physiological functions. It can slow your pulse and heart rate, lower your blood pressure, and decrease your levels of stress hormones. It can also help to reduce anxiety and induce sleep for women with cramps. Equally beneficial are types of nature sounds, such as ocean waves and rainfall, which can induce a sense of peace and relaxation. I have patients who keep tapes of nature sounds in their cars and at home for use when they feel more stressed. Play relaxing music often as your menstrual cycle approaches and you are aware of increased levels of emotional and physical tension.

Biofeedback Therapy

Biofeedback therapy is an effective way to relieve pain of all kinds caused by muscular tension, as well as poor circulation caused by narrowing of the blood vessel diameter. Constriction of the skeletal muscles and the smooth muscle of the blood vessel wall usually occurs on an unconscious basis, so a person is not even aware it's happening. A variety of factors, including emotional stress and nutritional and chemical imbalances, can trigger this involuntary muscle tension. This constriction can worsen problems such as migraine headaches, high blood pressure, and menstrual cramps.

Biofeedback therapy helps people recognize when they are tensing their muscles. Once this response is understood, menstrual cramp sufferers can learn to relax their muscles to relieve pain. Since muscle relaxation both decreases muscular discomfort and improves blood flow, either factor can be monitored. For relief of cramps, women learn how to implement biofeedback therapy through a series of training sessions. The series usually takes 10 to 15 half-hour office visits with a trained professional. During these sessions, a thermometer is inserted into the vagina like a tampon. The thermometer is connected to a digital readout machine that monitors the woman's internal temperature. The professional teaches her how to consciously change her vaginal temperature. Even a slight rise in the temperature indicates better blood flow and muscle relaxation in the pelvic area, with a concomitant relief of menstrual pain.

After the training sessions, most women are able to raise their temperature at will and thereby control their own cramps. I went through biofeedback training many years ago and found that it had a significant effect on my level of muscle tension. Many hospitals and university centers have biofeedback units, as do stress management clinics, so it is relatively easy to find a treatment facility that offers this type of therapy.

Putting Your Stress-Reduction Program Together

This chapter has introduced many different ways to reset your mind and body to help make menstruation a calm and relaxed time of the month. Try each exercise at least once. Experiment with them until you find the combination that works for you. Doing all seven exercises will take no longer than 20 to 30 minutes, depending on how much time you wish to spend with each one. Ideally, you should do the exercises at least a few minutes each day. Over time, they will help you to gain insight into your negative beliefs and change them into positive new ones. Your ability to cope with stress should improve tremendously.

8

Breathing Exercises for Menstrual Cramps

Therapeutic breathwork can have a major beneficial impact on menstrual cramps. Through the use of controlled breathing exercises, you can relax and loosen your muscles, decrease sensations of pain, lower your anxiety level, and generate a feeling of internal peace and calm.

When you are breathing slowly and deeply, you take in large amounts of oxygen from the environment. This oxygen is taken into your circulation where it binds to the red blood cells as it travels through the arteries and veins. Oxygen allows the cells to produce and utilize energy as well as help to remove waste products through the production of carbon dioxide. These waste products are cleared through exhalation by the lungs. Thus, the whole body needs optimal levels of oxygen for its normal cycle of building, repair, and elimination.

When you are in physical and emotional distress, oxygen levels are decreased. Breathing tends to become jagged, erratic, and shallow. You may find yourself breathing too fast or with severe pain. You may stop breathing altogether and hold your breath for prolonged periods of time without even realizing it. None of these breathing patterns is healthful. Anxious breathing is often linked to other unhealthy physiological reactions that reflect your body's state of stress.

When you have cramps, you tend to tense and tighten your muscles, constrict blood flow, elevate your pulse rate and heartbeat, and stimulate the output of stressful chemicals from your glands as a response to the pelvic discomfort. Waste products such as carbon dioxide and lactic acid also accumulate in your muscles and other tissues. Therapeutic breathing exercises provide a way to break up this pattern and help the body return to equilibrium. It is important to do the breathing exercises in a slow and regular manner and find a comfortable position.

Exercise 1: Deep Abdominal Breathing

Deep, slow abdominal breathing is a very important technique for the relief of menstrual cramps and pain. It brings adequate oxygen, the fuel for metabolic activity, to all tissues of the body. Rapid, shallow breathing decreases oxygen supply and keeps one devitalized. Deep breathing helps to relax the entire body, and strengthens muscles in the chest and abdomen. It also helps calm many other physiological processes, such as rapid pulse rate and heartbeat that often accompany menstrual cramps.

- Lie flat on your back with your knees pulled up. Keep your feet slightly apart. Try to breathe in and out through your nose.

- Inhale deeply. As you breathe in, allow your stomach to relax so that the air flows into your abdomen. Your stomach should balloon out as you breathe in. Visualize your lungs filling up with air so that your chest swells out.

- Imagine that the air you breathe is filling your body with energy.

- Exhale deeply. As you breathe out, let your stomach and chest collapse. Imagine the air being pushed out, first from your abdomen and then from your lungs.

Exercise 2: Peaceful, Slow Breathing

Breathing slowly and peacefully can actually decrease anxiety and help to promote a sense of inner calm and quiet. Such breathing helps our mind to slow down and our emotions to be happier and more harmonious. Life feels good. We make better decisions and relate to those around us in a healthier way when we are calm. Breathing slowly can also calm our physical responses by helping to balance autonomic nervous system function. The autonomic nervous system regulates functions that we're usually not aware of, such as circulation of the blood, muscle tension, pulse rate, breathing, and glandular function.

The autonomic nervous system is divided into two parts that oppose and complement each other, the sympathetic and parasympathetic systems. The sympathetic nervous system is linked to tension and the "fight or flight" response of fear and panic, while the parasympathetic nervous system regulates body responses that are relaxed and calm. When women have menstrual cramps and low back pain, the sympathetic nervous system is in overdrive. The pain sensation causes muscles to tense. Furthermore, the pulse rate tends to accelerate and the blood vessels tend to constrict. Slow, peaceful breathing is a way to calm down these stress responses and bring the body back to a state of balance. By slowing down our breathing, we slow down our other physiologic responses. Our muscles relax and our blood vessels dilate; a state of equilibrium is restored.

Lie flat on your back with your knees pulled up. Keep your feet slightly apart. Try to breathe in and out through your nose.

- Inhale deeply. As you breathe in, allow your stomach to relax so that the air flows into your abdomen. Let your stomach balloon out as you breathe in. Visualize the lowest parts of your lungs filling up with air.

- Imagine that the air you are breathing in is filled with peace and calm. A sensation of peacefulness and calm is filling every cell of your body. Your whole body feels warm and relaxed as you breathe in this air. Now, exhale deeply. As you breathe out, imagine the air being pushed out from the bottom of your lungs to the top.

- Repeat this sequence until your entire body feels relaxed and your breathing is slow and regular.

Exercise 3: Grounding

Women suffering from pain and discomfort due to fibroid tumors can lose a sense of being grounded, or rooted to the earth. Some women report a sensation of numbness in their legs and feet or feel as if they have no legs at all. The pelvic and low back pain resulting from menstrual cramps causes leg muscles to tighten and decreases blood circulation and oxygenation to lower extremities.

If you are feeling ungrounded focusing and concentrating can be difficult. You may have difficulty sitting at a desk and working through your projects for the day in a coherent manner. This exercise will help you to ground and focus both physically and mentally. You should feel much more stable and focused by the end of this exercise.

Sit upright in a chair. Be sure you are in a comfortable position. Keep your feet slightly apart. Breathe in and out through your nose.

- Inhale deeply. As you breathe in, allow your stomach to relax so that the air flows into your abdomen. Let your stomach balloon out as you breathe in. Visualize the lowest parts of your lungs filling up with air. Hold your inhalation.

- Visualize a golden cord with a golden ball at the end of it running from the base of your spine. Let this golden cord gently and slowly move downwards through the earth, grounding you. You can let it move down as far as you would like, even all the way to the center of the earth.

- Follow the cord and its golden ball in your mind all the way down and see it fasten securely to the earth's center. You can run two golden cords from the bottoms of your feet down to the center of the earth, also, if you would like.

- As you exhale, become aware of your hips, thighs, calves, ankles, and feet. Feel their strength and solidity.

Repeat this exercise several times until you feel fully present and grounded.

Exercise 4: Muscle Tension Release Breathing

This exercise will help you to get in touch with and release general muscle tension and tightness. Often when the uterus, abdominal muscles, and low back are tight, we unconsciously tense up muscles throughout the entire body. Often the neck, shoulders, and other vulnerable areas are tense, also. A woman with cramps can have tight and tense muscles in other parts of her body and not even be aware of it. This exercise will help you focus on any tension that you are carrying in your upper body. It will also help you take your focus off your cramps. As you relax and release the muscles in your neck and shoulders, it will help to release muscle tension in your entire body. This is also a good exercise to do while walking or doing sports or desk work, to get in touch with any muscle tension that you may be carrying.

- Sit upright in a chair. Be sure you are in a comfortable position. Keep your feet slightly apart. Try to breathe in and out through your nose.

- Inhale and exhale deeply. As you breathe, let your head move from side to side. Keep your shoulders down and try to touch your ear to your shoulder. As you do this movement, imagine that your neck is made out of putty and that it allows your head to move in a supple, relaxed movement from the left to the right. Now inhale and pull your shoulders up towards your ears.

- Hold your breath and keep your shoulders in a hunched position. Exhale and let your shoulders drop back into a relaxed, comfortable position. Repeat this several times.

- Inhale and exhale deeply as you roll your shoulders forward. Make a large, slow, circular motion with your shoulders. Then, roll your shoulders back slowly. Repeat this several times.

- Inhale and exhale deeply, keeping the rest of your body still and relaxed. Repeat this several times.

Exercise 5: Emotional Cleansing Breath

I have seen, during my years of medical practice, that muscle tension and pain is worse when women are under emotional stress. The more day-to-day stress that you have involving family, work, and other personal issues; the more this can negatively impact your menstrual cramps. In fact, many of my patients believe that their unhealed family and other personal relations, as well as sexual problems, are significant emotional triggers for their cramps and pain.

This exercise uses breathing to help you release any negative feelings, such as chronic anger or upset that you may be harboring. The more time you spend cleansing old negative emotional patterns, the less impact these feelings can have on your sensitive female reproductive tract with the onset of each menstruation.

- Lie flat on your back with your knees pulled up. Keep your feet slightly apart. Try to breathe in and out through your nose.

- Inhale deeply and see yourself enveloped in a soft white light. Breathe this light into every cell of your body. This is a cleansing light and can help wash away fear, anger, anxiety, and other negative feelings.

- As you exhale deeply, feel the light washing these emotions away.

- Repeat this exercise until you feel emotionally peaceful and clear.

Exercise 6: Color Breathing with Red and Blue

Color breathing has traditionally been used to heal the body and strengthen the body's energy field. Intuitives in our culture can see this energy field as light or colors emanating from the body. When a person is calm, relaxed, and healthy, the energy field appears radiant and full of colors. The colors are bright and harmonious, and each one corresponds to specific parts of the body.

When we are feeling pain or tension, which often happens with the chronic symptoms of endometriosis, we lose light and color. Our energy field looks more discordant and jagged, and often the colors change in response to the physical discomfort to duller, more muddied colors. Color breathing is a technique that can help strengthen and heal the energy field as well as the body itself. As you breathe in the healing colors, the parts of your body that are in pain and discomfort often begin to relax and feel healthier again. Tension and cramping is replaced by a sensation of lightness and peace.

- Sit or lie in a comfortable position.

- Take a deep breath and visualize that the earth below you is filled with a deep scarlet red color. This color goes 50 feet below you into the earth. Imagine that you are opening up energy centers on the bottom of your feet. See this color flowing in as you inhale; visualize the deep scarlet red color filling up your feet. Draw this color up your legs and into your pelvic area. See it first filling up your legs, then your lower back, and finally your pelvis. Your uterus is filling with a beautiful deep scarlet red color.

- As you exhale, see this color flow out of your uterus and lower back and fill the air around you. Exhale the deep scarlet red slowly out of your lungs. Repeat this process 5 times.

- Visualize that the earth is filled with a dark, inky, indigo blue. As you inhale, draw this color into the bottom of your feet. Let it fill your legs, lower back, and pelvic region. See this indigo blue color fill your uterus. As you exhale, see this color flow out of your uterus and lower back and fill the air around you. Exhale the deep indigo blue slowly out of your lungs. Repeat this process 5 times.

Exercise 7: Color Breathing with Golden Light

- Sit or lie in a comfortable position.

- Imagine a cloud of beautiful golden energy surrounding you. As you take a deep breath, inhale the golden energy and visualize it flowing through your body, into your uterus, pelvic area, and lower back. This is a healing energy—it warms and relaxes your uterus, lower abdominal muscles, and lower back.

- Hold the inhalation as long as it is comfortable. Let this golden cloud pick up all your pain and tension.

- Then, exhale this energy out through your lungs and be carried away from you.

- Repeat this process as many times as you need to, until the pain is replaced by a feeling of peace and calm.

9

Physical Exercise for Menstrual Cramps

During my teenage years and through my twenties, I had very few treatment options for my own menstrual cramps. The only treatments available to me were aspirin, heating pads, or bed rest. I often chose the latter and would lie, immobilized with pain, hoping my cramps would stop. During my internship year I began to learn about the importance of lifestyle intervention for the treatment and prevention of menstrual cramps. I began to increase my level of exercise and do more stretching and swimming. I also made significant changes in my dietary habits. Finally, after years of suffering, my menstrual cramps and low back pain started to disappear.

For a number of reasons, exercise promotes pain relief and prevention of menstrual cramps. When women are in pain, they tend to contract their muscles involuntarily. Tight and tense uterine and back muscles have decreased blood flow and oxygenation. Waste products such as excessive carbon dioxide accumulate in this physical environment and can further worsen symptoms. In addition, the pain of menstrual cramps causes breathing to become rapid and shallow. Less oxygen is taken in through respiration, which further decreases the oxygen available to the pelvic region. Metabolism of the muscles becomes less efficient, and fluid retention can become a problem in the pelvic area as well as the ankles and feet. Many women complain of aching pains in their thighs and aching sensations in their legs.

Vigorous aerobic exercise helps to relieve these symptoms of menstrual cramps. Exercise such as tennis, walking, swimming, and dancing requires deep breathing and active movement. Oxygenation and blood flow to the pelvic area improves with better respiration. The vigorous pumping action of the muscles that occurs with these activities helps to reduce the congestive symptoms of menstrual cramps by moving blood and other fluids from the pelvic region.

Exercise also produces significant psychological benefits to cramp sufferers. Improved oxygenation and blood flow benefit the brain as well as the pelvic muscles. The brain demands a healthy share of the body's available nutrients for optimal functioning. When the brain and nervous systems are functioning well, exercise helps to trigger an increased output of endorphins. These are chemicals made by the brain that have a natural opiate effect. Endorphins are thought to produce the "runner's high" that marathoners experience. Many women patients tell me that vigorous exercise is their most effective form of stress management; that exercise produces a sense of peace and relaxation unmatched by anything else they do.

Another way that aerobic exercise might help to reduce anxiety and calm the mood is by helping to balance the autonomic nervous system. The autonomic nervous system regulates the "fight or flight" response that many women experience around the time of their menstrual period. When this system is in overdrive, small life issues can become magnified out of proportion because the body reacts to these small stresses as if they were major life-threatening issues. Regular exercise helps to lessen the intensity of this response.

I also recommend that women with severe menstrual cramps and low back pain consider doing flexibility and stretching exercises as part of their physical activity program. These exercises help to prevent cramps and low back pain by strengthening the back and abdominal muscles. By balancing muscle tension through controlled, slow movement, stretching can also help to improve posture. Stretching exercises demand an awareness of how the parts of the body are aligned spatially with respect to the whole system when the exercises are done properly.

In summary, exercise brings many healthful benefits to women who suffer from menstrual cramps. I recommend that women with cramps follow a regular program of physical activity for cramps throughout the entire month, for both prevention and treatment of this condition. In many ways, exercise is the ideal medicine for women who suffer from menstrual cramps.

General Fitness and Flexibility Exercises for Menstrual Cramps

As part of your self-help program, the following exercises will promote mobility, flexibility, and relaxation. You can use them with great benefit during the premenstrual and menstrual time of the month to help loosen the joints in your lower body and decrease muscle stiffness and tension.

You can also do these exercises throughout the month. Practiced on a regular basis, they will improve your vigor and energy level. You can use them to warm up tense and tight muscles before engaging in sports or athletic events.

I do many of these exercises myself and have found them to be very helpful during times of physical and emotional stress and tension. They have helped me tremendously to stay loose and flexible with my own self-care program.

How to Perform the General Fitness and Flexibility Exercises for Menstrual Cramps

- Do all of these exercises during the first week or two of your program. Then put together your own routine based on the exercises that provide the most benefit. You may find that you want to use all of them on a regular basis, or perhaps only a few. Warm-ups should always precede any sports or athletic events.

- The exercises should be performed in a relaxed and unhurried manner. Be sure to set aside adequate time-30 minutes or more—so that you do not feel rushed. Your exercise area should be quiet, peaceful, and uncluttered.

- Wear loose, comfortable clothing. It is better to exercise without socks to give your feet complete freedom of movement and to prevent slipping.

- Wait at least two hours after eating to exercise. Evacuate your bowels or bladder before you begin the exercises.

- Choose a flat area and work on a mat or a blanket. This will make you more comfortable while you do the exercises.

- Pay close attention to the initial instructions when beginning an exercise. Look at the placement of the body as shown in the photographs. This is very important, for you are much more likely to have relief from your symptoms if you practice the exercise properly.

- Try to visualize the exercise in your mind, then follow with proper placement of the body.

- Move slowly through the exercise. This will help promote flexibility of the muscles and prevent injury.

- Always rest for a few minutes after doing the exercises.

- Try to practice these movements on a regular basis. A short session every day is best. If that is not possible, then try to practice them every other day.

Exercise 1: Joint Motion and Flexibility

When women are experiencing an episode of severe uterine cramping with the onset of menstruation, their first instinct is to simply curl up in the fetal position. Often a woman who has menstrual pain will simply stop moving or contract her breathing.

Immobilization is probably the worst thing you can do, because it further cuts off blood flow and oxygenation to the pelvic and low back areas, worsening the pain and tension. Gentle range of motion exercises help to loosen tense muscles where they insert and originate near the joints. The following sequence produces a gentle stretching of the muscles around the joints, which will help to reduce tension and stress. These stretches are also thought to stimulate the acupuncture meridians.

Sit on the floor with your legs stretched out in front. Place your hands at your sides.

Toes: Slowly flex and extend the toes without moving your feet or ankles. Repeat 10 times.

Ankles: Slowly flex and extend the ankle joints. Repeat 10 times. Separate your legs slightly, then rotate your ankles in each direction 10 times. Be sure to keep your heels on the floor.

Knees: Still resting in the sitting position, bend the right leg at the knee, bringing the heel near the right buttock. Then lift the right leg off the floor, straightening the right knee. Repeat 10 times. Then do the same exercise with the left leg.

Hold the thigh near the chest with both hands. Rotate your lower leg in a circular motion about the knee 10 times clockwise and then 10 times counterclockwise. Repeat with the left leg.

Hips: Bend the right leg so that you can place your right foot on the left thigh. Hold the right knee with the right hand and hold the right ankle with the left hand. Then gently move the right knee up and down with the right hand. Repeat with the left leg.

While you are sitting in the same position, rotate the right knee clockwise 10 times and then counterclockwise 10 times. This improves the flexibility of the hip joints. Repeat on the left side.

While sitting, bring the soles of the feet together, bringing the heels close to the body. Gently push the knees to the floor and then let them come up again. Repeat 10 times.

Spine: Remain sitting with your legs together straight out in front of you. Reach over and touch your legs or, without straining, your toes without bending your knees. Repeat 10 times.

Exercise 2: Muscle Tension Relaxation

This exercise set is excellent for releasing muscle tension and improving circulation in the lower body. It stretches the muscles in the pelvis and lower back. Many women who do this exercise also notice an increase in their energy level. You may have a feeling of vitality upon completing this sequence. The pelvic movements are particularly helpful in bringing optimal blood flow, oxygen, and nutrients to this region, which may help relieve cramps, low back pain, and abdominal tension. Do the steps slowly and never do them so hard as to cause a strain or injury.

Legs and Pelvis. Stand with your legs spread apart about two feet. Point your feet out at a comfortable angle. Bend your knees slowly and lower your buttocks. Eventually, they should be able to go as low as your knees. Move up and down 10 times. Then, rock your pelvis back and forth in a swinging motion.

Legs and Pelvis. Move your hips and pelvis from side to side. Let your torso and arms sway in the opposite direction, as if dancing. Then, move your hips around in a full circle. Do this several times in one direction and then the other.

Exercise 3: Lower Back Arch

This exercise helps loosen up the lower back muscles and promotes flexibility of the spine. It can also combat tiredness in women who experience deceased energy during the onset of menstruation.

Stand with your legs spread apart 1 foot. Point your feet straight ahead, place your hands around your waist with your thumbs pressing into your lower back.

As you inhale, curve your back into an arch with your head held back. Place your hands around your waist with your thumbs pressing into your lower back.

As you exhale, let the weight of your body bend you forward so that your head almost touches your knees. Hold for a few seconds. Do this exercise slowly and repeat several times.

Exercise 4: Abdominal Muscle Release

This exercise helps to release lower and upper abdominal tension. Many women with menstrual cramps often have digestive symptoms such as nausea and bowel changes. This twist helps to reduce the tension in the abdominal muscles that can worsen these symptoms.

Sit on the floor with your legs out in front. Place your hands on your shoulders with your fingers in front and thumbs in back. Be sure to keep your spine straight and inhale deeply.

As you inhale, twist your head, chest, and abdomen to the left. As you exhale, twist your body to the right.

Do this exercise 4 times, then reverse directions and repeat.

Exercise 5: Low Back Release

This exercise promotes relaxation, specifically in the lower back, hips, and abdominal muscles. By tensing and then releasing the abdominal and hip muscles, along with controlled heavy breathing, the entire mid- and lower body become looser and more supple. You may also notice a decrease in anxiety and emotional tension by the end of this exercise.

Lie on your back with your legs together.

Raise your feet 6 to 8 inches off the ground; then raise your head and shoulders 6 inches, also.

Point to your toes with your fingertips, keeping your arms straight and your eyes fixed on your toes. Then, breathe through your nose deeply to a count of 20.

Lower your legs and head and relax. Rest for a count of 30. Repeat this exercise several times.

Exercise 6: Low Back Twist

This exercise allows you to twist over to the side, which is actually a natural position for your body to assume when you are feeling pelvic discomfort. This gentle stretch helps to lengthen the muscles in the low back as well as along the entire spine. It also helps to align the lumbar spine. Many women find that this exercise helps relieve pelvic tension and discomfort.

Lie on your back with your knees bent, feet placed flat on the floor.

As you exhale, slowly let your knees and hips fall to the left as you turn your head to the right. Inhale and bring your knees back together to the center.

Then exhale again and reverse direction, letting your knees and hips fall to the right as you turn your head to the left.

Repeat this exercise slowly several times, alternating sides.

10

Stretches for Menstrual Cramps

Stretches can be tremendously beneficial in the treatment and prevention of menstrual cramps, pelvic congestion, and low back pain. The slow, controlled stretching movements that you do in these exercises help to relax tense muscles and improve their suppleness and flexibility. They also help to bring better blood circulation and oxygenation to the tense areas of your lower body, thereby improving the metabolism of the pelvic and back muscles. An additional benefit to stretches is that it helps to quiet your moods. The deep breathing and slow movement that accompany these exercises help to reduce anxiety and irritability and produce a sense of peace.

I have included a series of specific stretches poses that gently stretch every muscle in your body, with specific emphasis on the pelvic and low back region. As well as relieving cramps and discomfort, these exercises energize and balance the female reproductive tract and can help correct underlying hormonal imbalance through improved oxygenation and better circulation to the pelvic area. This can have a beneficial effect on menstrual function. Women who experience fatigue due to menstrual pain and discomfort can enjoy an increase in vigor and stamina when practicing the stretches exercises. I personally do stretches frequently as part of my own exercise routine.

When doing the exercises, it is important that you focus and concentrate on the positions. First your mind visualizes how the exercise is to look, and then your body follows with the correct placement of the pose. The exercises are done through slow, controlled stretching movements. This slowness allows you to have greater control over your body movements. You minimize the possibility of injury and maximize the benefit to the particular part of the body to which your attention is being directed.

Pay close attention to the initial instructions when beginning an exercise. Look at the placement of the body as shown in the photographs. This is very important, for if the pose is practiced properly, you are much more likely to have relief from your symptoms.

I would like to make the following suggestions as you begin these exercises: Try to visualize the pose in your mind, then follow with proper placement of the body. Move slowly through the pose. This will help promote flexibility of the muscles and prevent injury. Follow the breathing instructions provided in the exercise. Most important, do not hold your breath. Allow your breath to flow in and out easily and effortlessly.

If you practice these stretches regularly in a slow, unhurried fashion, you will gradually loosen your muscles, ligaments, and joints. You may be surprised at how supple you can become over time. If you experience any pain or discomfort, you have probably overreached your current ability and should immediately reduce the amount of the stretching until you can proceed without discomfort. Be careful, as muscular injuries can take quite a while to heal. If you do strain a muscle, I have found that immediately applying ice to the injured area for 10 minutes is quite helpful. Continue to use the ice pack two to three times a day for several days. If the pain persists, see your doctor.

Stretch 1

This exercise helps to relieve the low back tension that is so common with menstrual cramps. It also massages the neck and spine and flexes the vertebral column. It will invigorate and energize you, reducing fatigue. After doing this exercise, lie flat on your back for a few minutes to enhance the benefits of the exercise.

Lie on your back. Bend and raise your knees to your chest, clasping them with your hands. Hands should be interlocked below knees.

Raise your head toward your knees and gently rock back and forth on your curved spine. Note the roundness of your back and shoulders. Keep the chin tucked in as you roll back. Avoid rolling back too far on your neck. Rock back and forth 5 to 10 times.

Stretch 2

This is an excellent exercise for stretching the abdominal muscles which are often tightened with menstrual cramps. It is also helpful in reducing pelvic congestion.

Lie on your back with your knees bent. Spread your feet apart, flat on the floor.

Place your hands around your ankles, holding them firmly.

As you inhale, arch your pelvis up and hold for a few seconds. As you exhale, relax and lower your pelvis several times. Repeat this exercise several times.

Stretch 3

This exercise flexes the low back, strengthening this area. By building this area up over time, you can help to prevent menstrual cramps and low back pain.

Kneel on all fours. As you inhale, arch your spine downward while your head goes back.

As you exhale, curve your spine into a rounded arch while your head goes down. Do this exercise in a rhythmic, fluid manner.

Stretch 4

This exercise strengthens the back and abdominal muscles. It also improves blood circulation and oxygenation to the pelvis, which helps to decrease cramps and calms anxiety and nervousness.

Lie down and press the small of your back into the floor. This permits you to use your abdominal muscles without straining your lower back

Raise your right leg slowly while breathing in. Keep your back flat on the floor and let the rest of your body remain relaxed. Move your leg very slowly. Do not move your leg in a jerking manner. Hold for a few breaths.

Lower your leg and breathe out. Repeat the same exercise on your left side. Then alternate legs, repeating the exercise 5 to 10 times.

Stretch 5

This exercise strengthens the lower back, abdomen, buttocks, and legs and helps to prevent low back pain and menstrual cramps. It also energizes the entire female reproductive tract. Regular practice of this exercise helps to improve posture and elimination. It helps to reduce weight in the thighs and hips and tighten and firm the skin in these areas.

Lie face down on the floor. Make fists with both your hands and place them under your hips. This prevents compression of the lumbar spine while doing the exercise.

Straighten your body and raise your right leg with an upward thrust as high as you can, keeping your hips on your fists. Hold for 5 to 20 seconds if possible.

Lower the leg and slowly return to your original position. Repeat on the left side, then with both legs together. Remember to keep your hips resting on your fists. Repeat 10 times.

Stretch 6

This exercise stretches the entire spine and helps to relieve low back pain and menstrual cramps. It stretches the abdominal muscles and strengthens the back, hips, and thighs. It also stimulates the digestive organs and endocrine glands. Regular practice of this posture can help to relieve depression and fatigue, improving your energy and elevating your mood.

Lie face down on the floor, arms at your sides. Slowly bend your legs at the knees and bring your feet up toward your buttocks.

Reach back with your arms and carefully take hold of first one foot and then the other. Flex your feet to make grasping them easier.

Inhale and raise your trunk from the floor as far as possible. Lift your head and elevate your knees off the floor.

Squeeze the buttocks. Imagine your body looking like a gently curved bow. Hold for 10 to 15 seconds.

Slowly release the posture. Allow your chin to touch the floor and finally release your feet and return them slowly to the floor. Return to your original position. Repeat 5 times.

Stretch 7

This exercise also gently stretches the lower back. It is excellent for calming anxiety and irritability. This is one of the most effective exercises for relieving menstrual cramps.

Sit on your heels. Bring your forehead to the floor, stretching the spine as far over your head as possible.

Close your eyes. Hold for as long as this is comfortable.

Stretch 8

This exercise helps to relieve the congestive symptoms that occur with menstrual cramps. It opens the entire pelvic region and energizes the female reproductive tract. It also relieves bloating and fluid retention in legs and feet.

Lie on your back with your legs against the wall and extended out like a V or an arc, and your arms extended to the sides.

Hips should be as close to the wall as possible, buttocks on the floor. Legs should be spread apart as far as they can and still remain comfortable. Breathing easily, hold for 1 minute, allowing the inner thighs to relax.

Stretch 9

This exercise relieves menstrual cramps and low back pain. It also relieves anxiety and irritability and reduces eye tension and swelling of the face.

Lie on your back with a rolled towel placed under your knees. Your arms should be at your sides, palms up.

Close your eyes and relax your whole body. Inhale slowly, breathing from the diaphragm. As you inhale, visualize the energy in the air around you being drawn in through your entire body. Imagine that your body is porous and open like a sponge, so that this energy can be drawn in to revitalize every cell of your body.

Exhale slowly and deeply, allowing every ounce of tension to be drained from your body.

11

Acupressure for Menstrual Cramps

Acupressure massage is an ancient Chinese healing method that applies finger pressure to specific points on the skin surface to help prevent and treat illness. Acupressure has had a long and distinguished history as an effective healing tool for many centuries and is often used along with herbs to promote the healing of disease.

When specific acupressure points are pressed, they create changes on two levels. On the physical level, acupressure affects muscular tension, blood circulation, and other physiological parameters. On a more subtle level, Traditional Chinese Medicine believes that acupressure also helps to build the body's life energy to promote healing. In fact, acupressure is based on the belief that there exists within the body a life energy called chi. It is different from yet similar to electromagnetic energy. Health is thought to be a state in which the chi is equally distributed throughout the body and is present in sufficient amounts. It is thought to energize all the cells and tissues of the body.

The life energy is thought to run through the body in channels called meridians. When working in a healthy manner, these channels distribute the energy evenly throughout the body, sometimes on the surface of the skin and at times deep inside the body in the organs. Disease occurs when the energy flow in a meridian is blocked or stopped. As a result, the internal organs that correspond to the meridians can show symptoms of disease. The meridian flow can be corrected by stimulating the points on the skin surface. These points can be treated easily by hand massage. When the normal flow of energy through the body is resumed, the body is believed to heal itself spontaneously.

Stimulation of the acupressure points through finger pressure can be done by you or by a friend following simple instructions. It is safe, painless, and does not require the use of needles. It can be used without the years of specialized training needed for insertion of needles.

How to Perform Acupressure

Acupressure is done either by yourself or with a friend when you are relaxed. Your room should be warm and quiet. Make sure your hands are clean and nails trimmed (to avoid bruising yourself). If your hands are cold, put them under warm water.

Work on the side of the body that has the most discomfort. If both sides are equally uncomfortable, choose whichever one you want. Working on one side seems to relieve the symptoms on both sides. Energy or information seems to transfer from one side to the other.

Hold each point indicated in the exercise with a steady pressure for one to three minutes. Apply pressure slowly with the tips or balls of the fingers. It is best to place several fingers over the area of the point. If you feel resistance or tension in the area on which you are applying pressure, you may want to push a little harder. However, if your hand starts to feel tense or tired, lighten the pressure a bit. Make sure your hand is comfortable. The acupressure point may feel somewhat tender. This means the energy pathway or meridian is blocked.

During the treatment, the tenderness in the point should slowly go away. You may also have a subjective feeling of energy radiating from this point into the body. Many patients describe this sensation as very pleasant. Don't worry if you don't feel it—not everyone does. The main goal is relief from your symptoms.

Breathe gently while doing each exercise. The point that you are to hold is shown in the photograph accompanying the exercise. All of these points correspond to specific points on the acupressure meridians. You may massage the points once a day or more during the time that you have symptoms.

Acupressure Exercises

Exercise 1: Balances the Entire Reproductive System

This exercise balances the energy of the female reproductive tract and alleviates all menstrual complaints. It also helps relieve low back pain and abdominal discomfort.

Equipment: This exercise uses a knotted hand towel to put pressure on hard to reach areas of the back. Place the knotted towel on these points while your two hands are on other points. This increases your ability to unblock the energy pathways of your body.

Lie on the floor with your knees up. As you lie down, place the towel between the shoulder blades on your spine. Hold each step 1 to 3 minutes.

Cross your arms on your chest. Press your thumbs against the right and left inside upper arms.

Left hand holds point at the base of the sternum (breastbone).

Right hand holds point at the base of the head (at the junction of the spine and the skull).

Interlace your fingers. Place them below your breasts. Fingertips should press directly against the body.

Move the knotted towel along the spine to the waistline.

Left hand should be placed at the top of the pubic bone, pressing down. Right hand holds point on tailbone.

Exercise 2: Relieves Cramps, Bloating, Fluid Retention, Weight Gain

This sequence of points balances the points on the spleen meridian. It helps to relieve menstrual cramps. It also relieves bloating and fluid retention and helps to minimize weight gain in the period leading up to menstruation.

Sit up and prop your back against a chair, or lie down and put your lower legs on a chair. Hold each step for 1 to 3 minutes.

Left hand is placed in the crease of the groin where you bend your leg, one-third to one-half way between the hip bone and the outside edge of the pubic bone. Right hand holds a spot 2 to 3 inches above the knee.

Left hand remains in the crease of the groin. Right hand holds point below inner part of knee. To find the point, follow the curve of the bone just below the knee. Hold the underside of the curve with your fingers.

Left hand remains in the crease of the groin. Right hand holds the inside of the shin. To find this point, go four finger widths above the ankle bone. The point is just above the top finger.

Left hand remains in the crease of the groin. Right hand holds the edge of the instep. To find the point, follow the big toe bone up until you hit a knobby, prominent small bone.

Left hand remains in the crease of the groin. Right hand holds the big toe over the nail, front and back of the toe.

Exercise 3: Relieves Nausea

This exercise relieves the nausea and digestive symptoms that often occur with cramps and low back pain.

Lie on the floor or sit up. Hold these points 1 to 3 minutes.

Left index finger is placed in navel and pointed slightly toward the head. Right hand holds point at the base of the head.

Exercise 4: Relieves Menstrual Fatigue

This sequence of points relieves the fatigue that women experience just prior to the onset of their menstrual period. Tiredness may last through the first few days of menstruation for many women. This exercise can also help to relieve menstrual anxiety and depression. Caution: The second step in this sequence has traditionally been forbidden for use by pregnant women after their first trimester.

Sit up and prop your back against a chair. Hold each step for 1 to 3 minutes.

Left hand holds point at the base of the ball of the right foot. This point is located between the two pads of the foot.

Left hand holds the point midway between the inside of the right anklebone and the Achilles tendon. The Achilles tendon is located at the back of the ankle.

Left hand holds point below right knee. This point is located four finger-widths below the kneecap toward the outside of the shinbone. It is sensitive to the touch in many people.

Exercise 5: Relieves Low Back Pain and Cramps

This exercise relieves menstrual cramps and low back pain by balancing points on the bladder meridian. It also balances the energy of the female reproductive tract.

Sit on the floor and prop your back against a wall or a heavy piece of furniture. Hold each step for 1 to 3 minutes.

Alternative method: Lie on the floor and put your lower legs over the seat of a chair. Follow the exercise from that position.

Place left hand 1 inch above the waist on the muscle to the left side of the spine (muscle will feel firm and ropelike). Place right hand behind crease of the left knee.

Left hand stays in the same position. Right hand is placed on the center of the back of the left calf. This is just below the fullest part of the calf.

Left hand remains 1 inch above the waist on the muscle to the side of the spine. Right hand is placed just below the ankle bone on the outside of the left heel.

Left hand remains 1 inch above the waist on the muscle to the side of the spine. Right hand holds the front and back of the left little toe at the nail.

12

Treating Menstrual Cramps with Drugs

Women use several different types of medications to treat menstrual cramps. Some of these products can be bought over the counter, while other, stronger drugs need a doctor's prescription. Some medications—such as narcotics, diuretics, and muscle relaxants—have been around for a long time and have been the traditional treatments for cramps. Others, specifically the antiprostaglandins, have been widely available for use in treating menstrual cramps only for the past 15 years; these have provided women with a major source of symptom relief.

Over-the-Counter Medications

Many medications for menstrual cramp relief are available over the counter. They tend to be more effective for mild symptoms. My patients have reported to me over the years that these products usually don't provide sufficient relief of the more severe symptoms. One of the oldest cramp relief medications is simply aspirin. Interestingly enough, aspirin is a mild prostaglandin inhibitor, although it's only one-thirtieth as strong as the newer antiprostaglandin drugs. Always take aspirin with food to avoid stomach discomfort, and use it with great caution if you have a preexisting peptic ulcer or a tendency toward heartburn, because it can worsen or reactivate symptoms.

The F2 Alpha prostaglandins are hormone-like chemicals that cause uterine contractions when present in the reproductive tract in high concentrations around the time of menstruation. This can worsen menstrual pain and cramps. Always take aspirin with food to avoid stomach discomfort and use it with great caution if you have a preexisting peptic ulcer or a tendency toward heartburn, because it can worsen or reactivate symptoms.

Another prostaglandin inhibitor is ibuprofen. This drug is sold over the counter as Advil, Motrin or Nuprin, in 200 mg or 400 mg dosages. The dose commonly used for menstrual pain and cramps is two tablets, or 400 mg, taken every six hours. Aleve or naproxen sodium is also available as an OTC drug in a 220 mg dosage.

These medications are also available by prescription when taken in higher dosages. They include Motrin (in an 800 milligram dosage), Naprosyn or naproxen sodium as well as Ponstel. They tend to be very effective in relieving the symptoms of primary spasmodic dysmenorrhea and, for many women, can make the difference between being able to function during the menstrual period or being incapacitated by pain and spending one to two days in bed.

Antiprostaglandins are also used effectively to treat the pain symptoms in women with endometriosis, a common cause of secondary dysmenorrhea. These medications are particularly useful since they have both anti-inflammatory and painkilling activity.

These drugs must be used carefully, however, since they can cause gastrointestinal bleeding and peptic ulcer disease, or even reactivate a preexisting ulcer. Approximately 10 percent of women who use these medications report digestive symptoms. Symptoms including heartburn, nausea, vomiting, diarrhea, constipation, and poor digestion can occur as the result of using these medications.

To lessen the likelihood of these side effects, only take these medications with food and report any significant digestive symptoms to your physician. Some women report other uncomfortable symptoms when using prostaglandin inhibitors, such as drowsiness, headaches, vertigo, dizziness, rashes, blurred vision, anemia, edema, and heart palpitations. Avoid using these drugs with aspirin, since both can cause gastrointestinal bleeding and irritation.

Another group of over-the-counter remedies for menstrual pain contains several drugs used in combination. Products such as Midol, Pamprin, and a number of others on the market contain aspirin, an antispasmodic to relieve muscle tension, caffeine (which causes widening in the diameter of peripheral blood vessels), and sometimes a diuretic for relief of congestive symptoms. Be careful to follow the dosage instructions on the bottle; if used in excess, many of these drugs can cause undesired side effects. As mentioned earlier, aspirin can cause gastric distress.

Caffeine can make people nervous and jittery and may also upset the stomach by increasing gastric acid secretion. Diuretics can promote loss of minerals. Another commonly used ingredient in these products is pyrilamine, an antihistamine. Antihistamines are normally used to relieve symptoms of allergies such as nasal congestion. They also have as a side effect the tendency to cause drowsiness or sedation and are used in menstrual remedies for these sedative effects. Although the doses used are small, some women who are unusually sensitive may encounter side effects.

Prescription Medications

Narcotics. Narcotics such as codeine are very effective painkillers and can certainly numb the discomfort of menstrual cramps or endometriosis. They do, however, have significant side effects and don't reverse the underlying cause of the menstrual cramps or halt the spread of endometrial implants. These side effects commonly include constipation, nausea, and drowsiness. Be sure to avoid driving your car when using a significant painkiller because you may fall asleep at the wheel. Other painkillers like Darvon or relaxants like Valium are also prescribed. Although Valium is an effective relaxant, it can also cause drowsiness and sedation. All of these drugs can cause addiction. Women often find that higher doses and more frequent usage is needed to create a beneficial therapeutic effect if these drugs are used on a habitual basis.

I generally recommend that these drugs be used only on a very infrequent basis and only if symptoms are particularly severe.

Diuretics. Drugs such as HydroDiuril or Hygroton are strong medications usually prescribed to treat the fluid retention symptoms of primary congestive dysmenorrhea. Though diuretics help to relieve bloating and fluid weight gain by increasing fluid loss through the urinary tract, they also increase the loss of important minerals such as potassium and calcium from the body. Over time, potassium depletion can become a significant problem with frequent diuretic use. Side effects of potassium loss include weakness, fatigue, poor physical stamina, and muscle twitching and immobility. I used to see this problem much more commonly in the 1970s than now, since diuretic use has decreased with the advent of the new antiprostaglandin drugs. If you use any diuretic, be sure to increase your intake of fresh fruits, vegetables, and raw seeds and nuts, which are excellent sources of essential minerals. Eating a banana or two a day is particularly advised. It is easy to digest and contains a lot of potassium.

Birth Control Pills. These drugs prevent ovulation and thereby decrease the progesterone and prostaglandin accumulation during the second half of the menstrual cycle. This buildup of these two hormones has been associated with menstrual cramps. I recommend the birth control pills most strongly for women who wish to use this method as their primary form of contraception. Otherwise, a woman is using hormonal therapy all month to treat one or two days per month of menstrual cramp symptoms.

With endometriosis, however, the use of hormonal therapy has been an important treatment. Continuous hormonal therapy helps to relieve menstrual pain, however, it does not reverse the buildup of endometrial implants. There are women, however, who should avoid using birth control pills because of possible adverse side effects. These include women with a history of liver or gall bladder disease, migraine headaches, high blood pressure, and blood clots in the legs or pelvis. If you are interested in using the birth control pill, check with your physician to see if you are a good candidate.

Other Hormonal Therapies. Other hormonal therapies have also been used effectively to suppress estrogen and therefore menstruation. Two types of drugs are currently in use: synthetic steroids or hormones such as Danazol, and synthetic derivatives of the gonadotropin-releasing hormone (GnRH) such as Lupron. Danazol is a derivative of testosterone, the male hormone. It acts on the pituitary, the master endocrine gland, to inhibit hormonal output and suppress ovulation. Danazol is very effective in dissolving small endometrial implants and helps relieve symptoms in 85 percent of women who use it.

There are, however, significant drawbacks to its use. Twenty percent of women who take Danazol experience the recurrence of endometriosis symptoms within a year after stopping the drug. This percentage tends to increase with time. Danazol also causes masculinizing side effects such as acne, decrease in breast size, weight gain, oiliness of the skin and hair, deepening of the voice, and enlargement of the clitoris. Other side effects may be the same as those experienced in menopause due to the low levels of estrogen caused by the drug's therapeutic effects. These include hot flashes, increased sweating, and vaginal dryness. Obviously Danazol is a powerful drug that should be taken only after careful discussion between you and your physician.

Lupron, a commonly used gonadotropin releasing factor, is also an effective drug therapy for endometriosis. As many as 70 percent of women using Lupron or other drugs of this type note rapid symptom relief. Lupron is also used to shrink fibroid tumors. Unlike Danazol, Lupron does not cause masculinizing side effects, but does cause a marked pseudo-menopause because of significantly lowered estrogen levels. Like Danazol, Lupron can cause women to experience hot flashes, vaginal dryness, and a decrease in sex drive. Other side effects have included anemia, bone pain, nausea, vomiting, edema, low blood pressure, and sleep disorders. As with using Danazol, endometriosis symptoms may reoccur once the Lupron is stopped, just as they can reoccur after discontinuing Danazol. A woman can be back where she started before instituting the hormonal therapy.

If your secondary dysmenorrhea has another cause, such as pelvic inflammatory disease (PID), this situation must be treated in order to prevent recurrent pelvic pain. In this case, your physician should prescribe the appropriate antibiotic to destroy the infective agent. If drug therapy is unable to halt the severity of painful symptoms due to the structural damage and scarring that PID causes, a woman may need to undergo a complete hysterectomy to finally gain adequate pain relief.

Medications for Cramps

Over-the-Counter Medications
Aspirin
Ibuprofen (Advil, Nuprin)
Midol
Pamprin

Prescription Drugs

Antiprostaglandin Inhibitors
Motrin
Anaprox
Ponstel
Naprosyn

Narcotics
Codeine
Darvon

Relaxants
Valium

Diuretics
HydroDiuril
Hygroton

Hormonal Therapies
Birth control pills
Danazol
Lupron

13

How to Put Your Program Together

This book has given you a complete self-help program to help prevent and relieve your symptoms. The Complete Treatment Chart summarizes the many treatment options presented in this book. This chart should be very helpful to refer to as you put your own program together. Try the treatment options that feel most comfortable to you. You may find, for example, in trying the exercises or stress reduction techniques, that certain routines feel better to you than others. If that is the case, practice the ones that bring you the greatest sense of relief for your particular symptoms.

Don't get bogged down in details. Always keep in mind that your ultimate goal is relief of your menstrual cramps and a general improvement in your overall health and well-being. I generally recommend beginning any self-help program slowly so that you can get used to the lifestyle changes in a comfortable manner. People differ in their abilities to adjust to major life-style changes. Though some of my patients like to eliminate their old, unhealthy habits as quickly as possible, many other women find such rapid changes in their long-term habits to be too stressful. Find the pace that works for you.

Enjoy the program. I always tell my patients to regard their self-help program as an enjoyable adventure. The exercise and stress-reduction programs should give you a sense of energy and well-being. The menus and food selections I've recommended in this book provide you with an opportunity to try delicious and healthful new foods.

As you do the program, don't set up unrealistic or too strict expectations for yourself. You don't have to be perfect to get great results. Just follow the guidelines of the program as best you can and as your schedule permits.

It is not a disaster if you forget to take your vitamins occasionally or don't have time to exercise on any particular day. Don't be discouraged if you can't follow the dietary recommendations on vacations, holidays, and birthdays. Periodically, review the guidelines outlined in this book and continue to adapt your lifestyle to the healthful suggestions that I've shared with you from my years of medical practice. Over time you will notice many beneficial changes.

Be your own feedback system. Your own body will tell you if you are on the right track and if what you are doing is making you feel better. It will also tell you if your current diet and emotional stresses are worsening your symptoms. Remember that even moderate changes in your habits can make significant differences.

The Menstrual Cramps Workbook

Fill out the workbook section of this book. The workbook questionnaires will help you to evaluate which areas in your life have contributed the most to your symptoms and which areas need the most work. Use the workbook every month or two as you follow the self-help program. The workbook will help you to see the areas in which you are making the most progress, both with symptom relief and the initiation of healthier lifestyle habits. The workbook can help give you feedback in an organized and easy to use manner.

Diet and Nutritional Supplements

I recommend that you make all nutritional changes gradually. Many women find breakfast the easiest meal to change because it is simple and often eaten at home. To change your other meals and snacks, I recommend that you periodically review the list of foods to eliminate and foods to emphasize provided in this book. Each month pick a few foods that you are willing to eliminate from your diet. Try replacing them with the foods that help to prevent and relieve menstrual cramps, low back pain, and congestive symptoms. The recipes and menus that I've included in this book should be very helpful. The menus can provide you with helpful guidelines as you restructure your own needs.

Vitamins, minerals, and herbal supplements can help to complete your nutritional needs and speed up the healing process. For most women, they are a very important part of their program.

Stress-Reduction and Breathing Exercises

The stress-reduction and breathing exercises play an important role in facilitating the physical healing process. I find that all my patients heal more rapidly from almost any problem when they are calm, happy, and relaxed. Some of the exercises also provide a number of important visualizations that actually help you set a blueprint in your mind for optimal health. This allows the body and mind to work together in harmony.

Begin the program by putting 15 minutes to a half-hour aside each day, depending on the flexibility of your schedule. Try all the stress-reduction and breathing exercises listed in this book. Choose the combination that works best for you. Practice stress management on a regular basis and be aware of your habitual breathing patterns. Both of these techniques will help retrain your uterine, pelvic, and back muscles so that you can go through your period in a comfortable manner.

You do not need to spend enormous amounts of time on these exercises. Many women are too busy to spend an hour a day meditating. Even ten minutes out of your daily schedule can be helpful. You may find that the quietest times for you are early in the morning before you get out of bed and late at night before going to sleep. Other women simply choose to take a break during the day. You can close the door to your office or go into your bedroom at home for ten minutes to relax. Use the time to breathe deeply, do the visualizations, or meditate. You will be much calmer and more relaxed afterward.

Exercise

Moderate exercise should be done on a regular basis, at least three times a week. Aerobic exercise can help to improve both circulation and oxygenation to tight, constricted muscles, thereby helping you to relax. It is important, however, to do your exercise routine in a slow, comfortable manner. Frenetic exercise that is too fast-paced can push your muscles to the point of exhaustion and actually tense them further. It is important that women with menstrual cramps and low back pain keep their muscles and joints flexible and supple. Try the fitness and flexibility exercises in this book.

To do the stretches and acupressure exercises described in this book, I recommend that you set aside a half-hour each day for the first week or two of starting your self-help program. Try the exercises that appeal to you most. After an initial period of exploration, choose the ones that you enjoy and that seem to give you the most relief. Practice them on a regular basis so that they can help to prevent and reduce your symptoms.

Conclusion

I wish to reaffirm that each of us can do a tremendous amount for ourselves to assure optimal health and well-being. By having access to the all natural treatments in this book, you can play a major role in creating your own state of menstrual cramps-free good health. Practice the beneficial self-care techniques that I have outlined in this book. Follow good nutritional habits, exercise, and practice regular stress reduction techniques.

By combining good principles of self-care along with your regular medical care, you can enjoy the same wonderful results that my patients and I have had for a life of good health and well-being.

Love,

Dr. Susan

About Susan Richards, M.D.

Dr. Susan Richards is one of the foremost authorities in the fields of family medicine and alternative medicine. Dr. Richards has successfully treated many thousands of patients emphasizing alternative health and integrative medicine in her clinical practice. Her mission is to provide her patients with safe and effective alternative therapies to greatly enhance their health and well-being.

A graduate of Northwestern University Feinberg School of Medicine, she has served on the clinical faculty of Stanford University School of Medicine and taught in their Division of Family and Community Medicine.

Her Facebook page, Dr. Susan's Healthy Living, has over one million followers. She is also an ordained minister and her ministry receives over a million prayer requests for healing each year.

NOTES

NOTES

NOTES

References

(Athens). 2009 Jan-Mar;8(1):7-22. Review. http://hormones.gr/preview.php?c_id=503 (accessed 05/31/2011)

Balbi C, Musone R, Menditto A, et al., Influence of menstrual factors and dietary habits on menstrual pain in adolescence age. *EurJ Obstet Gynecol Reprod Biol.* 2000;91(2):143-8.

Barnard ND, Scialli AR, Hurlock D, Bertron P. Diet and sex-hormone binding globulin, dysmenorrhea, and premenstrual symptoms. *Obstet Gynecol.* 2000;95(2):245-50.

Blommers J, de Lange-De Klerk ES, Kuik DJ, et al. Evening primrose oil and fish oil for severe chronic mastalgia: a randomized, double-blind, controlled trial. Am J Obstet Gynecol 2002;187:1389-94.

Budeiri D, Li Wan Po A, Doman JC. Is evening primrose oil of value in the treatment of premenstrual syndrome? Control Clin Trials 1996;17:60-9.

Casper RF, et al. Clinical manifestations and diagnosis of premenstrual syndrome and premenstrual dysphoric disorder. http://www.uptodate.com/home/index.html. Accessed May 20, 2010.

Casper RF, et al. Treatment of premenstrual syndrome and premenstrual dysphoric disorder. http://www.uptodate.com/homefindex.html. Accessed May 20, 2010.

Chasteberry. Natural Medicines Comprehensive Database. http://www.naturaldatabase.com. Accessed June 16, 2010.

Chen HM, Chen CH. Effects of acupressure t the Sanyinjiao point on primary dysmenorrhea. JAdv Nurs. 48.4 (2004):380-387

Cheung K. Management of cyclical mastalgia in oriental women: pioneer experience of using gamolenic acid (Efamast) in Asia. Aust NZJ Surg 1999;69:492-4.

Combs, G.F. *The Vitamins: Fundamental Aspects in Nutrition and Health.* 2008. San Diego: Elsevier.

Comparison of fennel and mefenamic acid for the treatment of primary dysmenorrhea. Int J Gynaecol Obstet. 2003.

Dennehy CE. The use of herbs and dietary supplements in gynecology: an evidence-based review. J Midwifery Womens Health. 51.6 (2006):402-409.

Dennehy CE. The use of herbs and dietary supplements in gynecology: an evidence-based review. *J Midwifery Womens Health.* 2006;51(6):402-9. Fjerbaek A, Knudsen **UB**. Endometriosis, dysmenorrhea and diet -- what is the evidence? *Eur J Obstet Gynecol Reprod Biol.* 2007;132(2):140-7.

Epel ES. Psychological and metabolic stress: a recipe for accelerated cellular aging? *Hormones*

Facchinetti F, Borella P, Sances G, Fioroni L, Nappi RE, Genazzani AR. Oral magnesium successfully relieves premenstrual mood changes. *Obstet Gynecol.* 1991;78:177-181. http://www.ncbi.nlm.nih.gov/pubmed/2067759 (accessed 05/23/2011)

Fjerbaek A, Knudsen UB. Endometriosis, dysmenorrhea and diet-What is the vidence? Eur J Obstet Gynecol Reprod Biol. 2007 jan 6.

French L. Dysmenorrhea. Am Fam Physocoan. 71.2 (2005) 285-291.

Gold CE, at al. Diet and lifestyle factors associated with premenstrual symptoms in a racially diverse community sample: Study of Women's Health Across the Nation (SWAN). Journal of Women's Health. 2007;16:541.

Grimes DA, Hubacher D, Lopez LM, Schulz KF. Non-steroidal anti-inflammatory drugs for heavy bleeding or pain associated with intrauterine-device use. *Cochrane Database Syst Rev.* 2006;(4):CD006034.

Guerrera MP, Volpe SL, Mao JJ. Therapeutic uses of magnesium. *Am Fam Physician.* 2009 Jul 15;80(2):157-62. Review.

Habek D, Cortez Habek J, Bobic-Vukovic M, Vujic B. Efficacy of acupuncture for the treatment of primary dysmenorrheal. *Gynakol Geburtshiffliche Rundsch.* 2003 Oct;43(4):250-253.

Hardy ML. Herbs of special interest to women. J Am Pharm Assoc (Wash). 2000 Mar-Apr;40(2):234- 42; quiz 327-9. http://www.ncbi.nlm.nih.gov/pubmed/10730024 (accessed 05/31/2011).

Harel z, Biro FM, Kottenhahn RK, Rosenthal SL. Supplementation with omega-3 polyunssaturated fatty acids in the management of dysmenorrhea in adolescents. Am J Obstet Gynecol. 174.4 (1996): 1335-1338.

Huang HY, Caballero B, Chang S, et al. Multivitamin/mineral supplements and prevention of chronic disease: executive summary. *Am J Clin Nutr.* 2007;85:265S. http://www.ajcn.org/content/85/1/265S.short (accessed 05/23/2011)

J Altern Complement Med. 2009. Comparison of effects of ginger, mefenamic acid, and ibuprofen on pain in women with primary dysmenorrhea. Shahid Beheshti University of Medical Sciences, Tehran, Iran.

Kashanian M, Mazinani R, Jalalmanesh S. Pyridoxine (vitamin B6) therapy for premenstrual syndrome. *Int J Gynaecol Obstet.* 2007;96:43-44. (No abstract available.)

Khoo SK, Munro C, Battistutta D. Evening primrose oil and treatment of premenstrual syndrome. Med J Aust 1990;153:189-92.

Kidd PM. Omega-3 DHA and EPA for cognition, behavior, and mood: clinical findings and structural-functional synergies with cell membrane phospholipids. *Altern Med Rev.* 2007 Sep;12(3):207-27. 3 http://www.altmedrev.com/publications/12/3/207.pdf (accessed 05/31/2011).

Koseoglu E, Talaslioglu A, Gontil AS, Kula M. The effects of magnesium prophylaxis in migraine without aura. *Magnes Res.* 2008;21:101-108. http://www.ncbi.nlm.nih.gov/pubmed/18705538 (accessed 05/23/2011)

Letzel H, Megard Y, Lamarca R, Raber A, Fortea J. The efficacy and safety of aceclofenac versus placebo and naproxen in women with primary dysmenorrhea *Eur J Obstet Gynecol Reprod Biol.* 2006;129(2):162-8.

Lloyd KB, Hornsby LB. Complementary and alternative medications for women's health issues. *Nutr C/in Pract.* 2009 Oct-Nov;24(5):589-606

Nagata C, Hirokawa K, Shimizu N, Shimizu H. Associations of menstrual pain with intakes of soy, fat and dietary fiber in Japanese women. *EurJ C/in Nutr.* 2005;59(1):88-92.

Pouresmail Z, Ibrahimzadeh R. Effects of acupressure and ibuprofen on the severity of dysmenorrheal. *J Tradit Chin Med* 2002 Sep;22(3):205-210.

Proctor ML, Hing W, Johnson TC, Murphy PA. Spinal manipulation for primary and secondary dysmenorrhea. *Cochrane Database Syst Rev.* 2006;3:CD00211..

Proctor ML, Latthe **PM,** Farquhar CM, Khan KS, Johnson NP. Surgical interruption of pelvic nerve pathways for primary and secondary dysmenorrhea. *Cochra, Database Syst Rev.* 2005 Oct 19; (4):CD001896.

Proctor ML, Murphy PA, Pattison **HM,** Suckling J, Farquhar CM. Behavioural interventions for primary and secondary dysmenorrhea. *Cochrane Database Syst Rev.* 2007;(3):CD002248.

Pye JK, Mansel RE, Hughes L.E. Clinical experience of drug treatments formastalgia. Lancet 1985;2:373-7.

Sayegh R, et al. The effect of a carbohydrate-rich beverage on mood, appetite, and ognitive function in women with premenstrual syndrome. Obstetrics & Gynecology. 1995;86:520.

Schellenberg R. Treatment for the premenstrual syndrome with agnus castus fruit extract: prospective, randomised, placebo controlled study. *BMJ.* 2001;322:134.

Thys-Jacobs S, Starkey P, Bernstein D, Tian J. Calcium carbonate and the premenstrual syndrome: effects on premenstrual and menstrual symptoms. Premenstrual Syndrome Study Group. *Am J Obstet Gynecol.* 1998;179:444-452. http://www.ncbi.nlm.nih.gov/pubmed/9731851 (accessed 05/23/11)

Tugay N, Akbayrak T, Demirturk F, et al. Effectiveness of transcutaneous electrical nerve stimulation and interferential current in primary dysmenorrhea. *Pai Med.* 2007;8(4):295-300.

Walker AF, De Souza MC, Vickers MF, Abeyasekera S, Collins ML, Trinca LA. Magnesium supplementation alleviates premenstrual symptoms of fluid retention. *J Womens Health.* 1998;7:1157 1165. http://wwvv.ncbi.nlm.nih.gov/pubmed/9861593 (accessed 05/23/2011)

Wang P, Ren J, Tang J, Zhang D, Li B, Li Y. Estrogen-like activities of saikosaponind in vitro: a pilot study. *Eur J PharmacoL* 2010 Jan 25;626(2-3):159-65. Epub 2009 Oct 9. http://www.ncbi.nlm.nih.gov/pubmed/19819234 (accessed 05/31/2011).

Whelan AM, Jurgens TM, Naylor H. Herbs, vitamins and minerals in the treatment of premenstrual syndrome: a systematic review. *Can J Clin Pharmacol.* 2009 Fall;16(3):e407-29. Epub 2009 Oct 29. http://www.ncbi.nlm.nih.gov/pubmed/19923637 (accessed 05/31/2011)

Wong CL, Farquhar C, Roberts H, Proctor M. Oral contraceptive pill for primary dysmenorrhoea. *Cochrane Database Syst Rev.* 2009 Oct 7;(4):CD002120.

Wuttke W, Jarry H, Christoffel V, Spengler B, Seidlova-Wuttke D. Chaste tree (Vitex agnus-castus)— pharmacology and clinical indications. *Phytomedicine.* 2003 May;10(4):348-57. https://wwvv.ncbi.nlm.nih.gov/pubmed/12809367 (accessed 05/31/2011).

Wyatt KM, Dimmock PW, Jones PW, Shaughn O'Brien PM. Efficacy of vitamin B-6 in the treatment of premenstrual syndrome: systematic review. *BMJ.* 1999 May 22;318(7195):1375-81. https://www.ncbi.nlm.nih.go /PMC27878/ (accessed 05/31/2011)